This is a truly amazing work and telling the many stories of the human soul, of the depth of the human spirit and the power of unconditional love! These stories are so close to the heart, I cannot imagine anything else giving students and caregivers an idea of the core of our elder communities. Through Mary Ann's stories, we discover that elders of any age and in any condition—especially forgetful (also disparagingly called: demented)—belong to the wisest and most loving of beings our community of humans has created. Mary Ann shows this hardly known fact like few other writers ever have. A must read for those of us in fear of aging and becoming frail, fragile and dependent.

—Nader Shabahangi, Ph.D., Founder of Pacific Institute and AgeSong, Co-author, *Conversations with Ed*

Ms. Konarzewski embodies a rare combination, that of a gifted writer and that of a deeply compassionate caregiver. She has a gift for storytelling that not only brings alive her characters, but also her inner experience as a care provider who draws from a deep spiritual source as she cares from the heart. One cannot help but see the author's clients through her eyes, as loveable and precious even with their foibles, limitations, and shadows. There is an infectious enthusiasm in Ms. Konarzewski that makes us enjoy, against all expectation, the events she describes about life in care homes. We are inspired as we listen to the author tell us how she gently encourages new adventures in the lives of her octogenarian clients. The result is reclaiming neglected gifts, healing family relationships, and increased joy among fellow long-term care residents.

—Rev. Jurgen Schwing, M.A. BCC Director Spiritual Care Services, Kaiser Permanente Diablo Service Area

Mary Ann Konarzewski has cleared a master path rooted in the wisdom of the heart so that anyone who loves and cares for frail elders can become more adept. She lays down a vision: opens the heart with stories about how the vison can be made manifest; and then describes steps we can take to advance on the path of sacred service. Her imaginative, bold humility provides the illumination.

—Barry Barkan, Ashoka fellow recipient,
Co-founder of Life Oak Institute and Elders Guild

Ms. Konarzewski provides a model for elder care that deserves attention, praise, and emulation.

—Stanley Krippner, Ph.D., Professor of Psychology
and Humanistic Studies, Saybrook University,
Co-author of *The Mythic Path and Healing Stories*

Mary Ann shows us the essential humanity of every elder in the book and shows us how to love elders with an open heart and questioning mind. We learn how to interact with elders as sentient beings worthy of kindness and respect, no matter their diagnosis or behavior. We also learn how important it is for elders to be heard and seen, how they are capable of growth and change, and how elders living in care homes want to be assisted according to their individual needs, not those of the institution. Mary Ann has given us a gem of a book. I cannot wait to add it to my library.

—Debora Barkan, Co-founder of the
Live Oak Institute and Elders Guild

Creating a Rich and Meaningful Life in Long-Term Care is, truly, about love. Mary Ann has the gift of giving and receiving. She gives us beautiful stories with helpful recommendations that focus on quality interactions during challenging transitions in life. This book is a great tool and must read for anyone in a caregiving role, those who work with elders and students. Thank you Mary Ann for pairing your memoirs with thoughtful and useful activities."

—Dr. Katerina Rozakis, Ph.D., LCSW,
DAPA, BCIM, Founder of Insight for Wellness

CREATING A RICH AND MEANINGFUL LIFE IN LONG-TERM CARE

A Guide for Family Caregivers and Elder Care Professionals

by
Mary Ann Konarzewski

Apocryphile Press
1700 Shattuck Ave #81
Berkeley, CA 94709
www.apocryphile.org

© Copyright 2017 by Mary Ann Konarzewski
Printed in the United States of America

ISBN 978-1-944769-82-6

These stories portray real people and events, but the names and some circumstantial details have been changed to protect privacy.

Please join our mailing list at
www.apocryphilepress.com/free
and we'll keep you up-to-date on all our new releases
—and we'll also send you a FREE BOOK. Visit us today!

CREATING A RICH AND MEANINGFUL LIFE IN LONG-TERM CARE

A Guide for Family Caregivers
and Elder Care Professionals

For my mother, husband, and all the elders
whose lives have touched mine.

ACKNOWLEDGMENTS

I am deeply grateful to my beloved husband, Charles Burack, who for years has encouraged me to write this book. I am grateful for his invaluable insights and suggestions and the time he spent reviewing and editing the manuscript. Were it not for his ever present support and inspiration, this book would not have been born. He made fertile the ground through which it was created. His love, wisdom, and playful humor continually nurture me and keep me going.

I am grateful to John Mabry at Apocryphile Press for his enthusiasm, wisdom, and expansive vision. Without his suggestions and guidance, this book would never have developed into its current form. He has been a true angel and guiding light.

To Katerina Rozakis-Trani, founder of Insight for Wellness Center, for her encouragement and support from the very beginning. Her integrative approach to health and wellness, her wisdom, loving presence, big heart, and entrepreneurial spirit have been a source of light and inspiration. I appreciate the time she devoted to reviewing my manuscript.

To Laura L. Benn, founder of Guided Health Care, for her enthusiastic support, keen insight, and lively spirit, for her dedication to the elders and families she serves and for her embracing a larger vision committed to healing and transformative change.

I am grateful to my dear friend Monica Englander for the depth and breadth of her mind, her listening heart, and for

1

teaching me how to "see." Her ever loving friendship, presence, and support continually nourish and inspire me.

To Barry and Debora Barkan, visionaries and pioneers in the field of elder care, and founders of the Life Oak Institute and Elders Guild. I began my career at Life Oak Institute, not knowing whether this work was my calling. Being a part of Live Oak confirmed that it was. A door was opened, a seed was planted and started to sprout. Their enthusiastic support means much to me. Special thanks to Barry for his powerful blessing nearly two decades ago which continues to ripple out into my life and the lives of the elders I touch. Special thanks to Debora for her helpful and inspiring suggestions regarding the manuscript.

I am grateful to the staff at the Reutlinger Community with special thanks to Caroline Allen, LCSW, Director of Social Services, for her unrelenting determination and commitment to creating healing and transformative change within the lives of the individual elders and communities she serves.

To Carol Goldman, Director of Life Enrichment at the Reutlinger Community, who allowed me the freedom to create programs that were "outside the box," many of which are illustrated in this book.

To Betty Rothaus, Art Program Director/Artist-in-Residence at the Reutlinger Community, for the wisdom, beauty, and passion she brings to her work with elders and the sacred space she has created for her students to paint, draw, dream, imagine, and create. She has taught me about how art can heal and transform, create connection and bring deeper meaning.

To the staff at Moraga Post-Acute Care, formerly known as Grace Healthcare, with special thanks to Elizabeth Lukacsy, former Activity Director at Grace Healthcare; Molly Jones, former Administrator; Nabeta Kisajja, former Director of Nursing; Kate Elliott, former Activity Director; Bali Johal, former Unit Manager; Ben Pyper, Administrator of Moraga Post-Acute Care; Mona Silveira, Activity Director; Nicole Long, Nurse Practionor;

Maria Pulido, RNA; Lauretica Randle, CNA; and Shashi Kumar, CNA.

To MoMa for the inspiration they gave me through their art program for people living with dementia, and for their generosity in sending me their books and materials at no cost and allowing me the time to ask questions.

To Stanley Krippner, pioneering psychologist and prolific author, for the time he spent reviewing my manuscript. He has been an inspiration in illuminating the power and magic of dreams.

To Nader Shabahangi, author, founder and CEO of AgeSong assisted living, for his enthusiastic support of my book and the time he spent reviewing it. His pioneering vision of aging and elder communities has been a source of light and inspiration.

To Irene Kessel, for her collaborative spirit and for teaching me about the power of music to heal and create community. To Christie Gough for her enthusiastic interest in reading my manuscript and for her encouragement and support. I appreciate the time she spent reviewing it.

To Karen Kelleher, Dementia Coordinator at St. Paul's Towers for her enthusiastic support and for making herself available to me on numerous occasions to share her thoughts and ideas on elder care, culture change, and semantics. I greatly value our conversations.

To Mark Witte, Program Director, emeritus at St. Paul's Towers, and Dyke Brown, founder of the Athenian School, who was a resident at St. Paul's Towers. To Annelisa Schinzinger and my beloved friend Ernest Thalinger, whose blessed memory lives on within me.

I am grateful to the staff at Atria Valley View, with special thanks to Juliana Munroe, Engage Life Director, and Lydia Swagerty, former Engage Life Director; and the staff at Byron Park with special thanks to Kate Geraghty, Engage Life Director.

To Lauren Eppinger, LCSW at Advisors on Aging, and to Diana Lowe, Janice Kitteridge, and Jill Judson, Fiduciaries at Senior Connection.

To Rosemary Lum-Levine and her husband, Michael Lisman, for their ever loving presence and friendship, for their enthusiastic support and encouragement in my bringing this book into the world.

To Jurgen and Debra Schwing for their loving presence and support. I appreciate the time Jurgen spent in carefully reviewing my manuscript.

To Mike Lane for being such a great listener and cheerleader for me and for everyone else he loves.

To Ralph Dranow for his enthusiastic support of the book and his valuable edits. And to Naomi Rose, his wife, for her loving friendship, support, and encouragement.

To Priscilla Buchman for her enthusiastic encouragement and support of the book, her big heart, and playful humor.

To Raphael Rettner for his enthusiasm over the stories I once shared at our dinner table, and for his urging me to write a book. To Colette de Gagnier-Rettner, my Tagore-loving Indian soul sister, for the beauty and inspiration she brings to my life, and for showing me how to use Facebook and create a page for this book.

To Pat Sullivan for her enthusiastic support of the book and astute editing and proofreading in the book's final stage. She offered many helpful suggestions and always made herself available whenever I had a question.

To Mary and John Laird for their loving support throughout the years with special thanks to Mary for the inspiration, beauty, and wisdom she brings to my life. She is an angel divine under whose wing I have blossomed.

To my mother-in-law, Ruth Burack, for her loving support and care for my wellbeing. With eager ear, she always listened and encouraged me in my work with elders.

To my mama, whose ever loving spirit and presence continues to live within me, gently encouraging, loving and guiding me, and making me smile. She has been one of my greatest teachers and heroes!

To my papa and the many blessings he gave me. He taught me about kindness and the meaning of god and the impermanence of life. His love will always live within me, and his guidance continues to be heard in the silence of my heart.

To my great octogenarian uncle, Fufu, and the gift he gave me of understanding what it means to grow old in a culture that honors youth and sometimes tries to forget or hide our elders. He taught me about patience, kindness, compassion, and planted the seed of what would become one of my life callings.

To my brother whom I can see beaming down from the heavens with his ever protective gaze, and caring, loving presence.

And I want to give thanks to all the elders and their families whose lives have touched mine. Some of their stories are in this book. Special thanks to all the caregivers who continually toil to make the lives of the elders better.

Finally, I want to thank all my friends and colleagues whose names I have not mentioned, you all make a difference in my life and work.

CONTENTS

PART VIII
SURRENDERING TO
THE FLOW OF THE SEASONS

PART IX
THE BITTERSWEET TRANSIENCE OF LIFE

PART X
PLAY, PRESENCE, LAUGHTER AND JOY

PART XI
SEEING BEYOND THE ANGER

PART XII
WHEN THE SUN GOES DOWN

PART XIII
IN THE END, IT'S ALL
ABOUT LOVE AND ONLY LOVE

APPENDIX

PART I

IN THE BEGINNING
IT'S ALL ABOUT LOVE...

INTRODUCTION

For nearly two decades I have worked with elders in long-term care as a social service worker, activity director, activity therapist, consultant, and certified massage therapist. I have had many heartfelt and inspired relationships with the elders I've served. Many have had dementia, Alzheimer's, Parkinson's, or a host of other conditions that limit the full functioning of the mind or body. Some have been completely lucid yet unable to physically manage on their own.

In spite of these limitations, many have continued to live long, productive lives, devoting their time to discovering hidden talents and gifts. I have seen elders blossom and live out long, cherished dreams. I have also watched elders dwindle when neglected by family and friends and not given the opportunity for continued growth.

Each elder I have written about is a living treasure, a legacy within my heart. They have all touched me deeply. I hope that their stories will touch and inspire you, too.

This book is for anyone who is actively involved in elders' lives: family members, eldercare professionals, clinicians, friends, and volunteers working with elders. My hope is that these stories will spark within you new ways of relating to the elders in your life that will make their lives better, richer, and more meaningful. I hope you will be encouraged to not give up on your loved ones, no matter how disoriented, non-communicative, or remote they may seem. I hope too that you will take away new insights into what many elders experience as they grow older in a care setting, and what you can do to help.

Each chapter begins with one or more essential key points, which are then illustrated in the story. Ideas for creating engaging and inspiring activities, as well as tips and further thoughts are provided at the end of many of the stories. All suggested activities can be easily adapted for family caregivers, as well as activity directors and other elder care professionals. If you are a family caregiver, and an idea inspires you but involves a community, I encourage you to talk to the activity director at your community or to other elder care professionals assisting you. Share the story and your thoughts about what you would like to do, and make it a collaboration.

At the back of this book, you will find three appendices. The first contains information specific to people with Alzheimer's. The second summarizes the gifts and lessons I've gathered in my journey with these elders. The third concludes with suggested readings and resources. Feel free to jump around in the book, choosing the chapters or sections which interest you most.

Among the 43 stories in this book, you will meet Bee, who at 85 years old becomes a painter. By "communing with Spirit," as she describes it, Bee is able to work with her paint and canvass to create masterpieces so exquisite that they have been exhibited in museums. Her life is one of constant creation and imagination in spite of not being able to walk and having to rely on caregivers 24/7.

And you will meet Rodger, who at the tender age of 65, was put on hospice with a brain tumor and three months to live. But when those three months were up, quite miraculously, he was taken off hospice because he kept getting better. For the first time in his life, he had fallen in love — with a feisty woman 25 years his senior.

And there is Emma, who at 85, has Alzheimer's, and is one of my greatest teachers. She inspires me to ponder the world and how much more peace there might be if, like her, we knew how to love without judging — seeing the beauty and wonder within each and every being. Every day she rushes towards me with a big smile to embrace me and say, "I love you. You are so wonderful." With her effervescent blue eyes, she takes me in. We have not known each other for very long, but with a warmth and affection that mirrors hers, I embrace her and tell her the same. That is the extent of our conversation, yet I look forward to our hugs and our intimate exchange of words. They add something special and uplifting to my day.

And there is Rosie, who at 99 years old, suddenly found herself in skilled nursing for the first time in her life because of a broken hip. "What am I doing here with all these old people? I don't belong here!" she whispered in my ear while staring through her goggle-like glasses at the other elders, who, like her, were all in wheelchairs, except she was so tiny that her feet barely touched the floor.

She then looked at me and waited for my reply. Charmed and touched by her, I threw my arms around her and said, "I love you, Rosie."

She smiled back and said, "Hey, maybe I am here so we could get to know each other." From that moment, Rosie captured my heart, and I began visiting her every day.

One day Rosie said to me, "Don't forget to put me in that book of yours."

"What book?" I asked.

"The one you are writing about all these people in here."

I was puzzled because writing a book about *all these people in here* was the furthest thing from my mind. I had no such intention.

My writing this book and my working with elders both came about unexpectedly, serendipitously, yet I could not imagine my life having passed without having done either one. Both experiences have held some of the most inspired and wondrous moments in my life, moments in which I felt there must be something bigger and greater that propels and moves all things into being—the spirit of love.

This book is about the power and beauty of love. It is about accepting the changes in our loved ones as they age, and seeing what is still possible, instead of focusing on what is no longer possible. Many of these stories are about how the creative arts can be used with elders, including the transformative affects the arts can have on people with dementia. Through poetry, storytelling, and painting, the self is recognized and nurtured.

My work with elders was inspired by my mother, who over fifteen years ago was suddenly diagnosed with terminal cancer. I returned home to take care of her during the last few months of her life. Although I had lost many people in my life–my father, my brother and a best friend, I had never been with anyone while they were dying, much less taken care of anyone in their final days. Being the only family member left, I was alone, sad, and frightened. Yet as the days passed, I began to feel the power of a bigger presence and no longer felt lonely or afraid. It was one of the most profound and transformative experiences in my life: a true gift.

Whatever petty worries and concerns I had paled in comparison to this: my mother was about to embark on one of the most important journeys one can possibly take in this lifetime. She would be leaving all this behind: her daughter, her possessions, and her body.

I was there to help prepare her for that journey. I was there to do whatever was required of me: to take care of her needs and last wishes; to help ease her pain and suffering; and to make her as comfortable as possible. I would sit with an open heart and be deeply present to her. I would try to create an atmosphere of complete love, peace, forgiveness, nurturance, and healing.

Death was nearing, and I could feel it. Yet what I experienced wasn't death as an ending but as a continuation of a greater life. The presence of that greater life filled the room. I no longer felt like I was taking care of my mother. Rather, that larger force was moving through me as I bathed her, fed her, lay next to her, massaged her, tended to her business, answered her calls and visits, sat in silence with her, prayed with her, held her hand, and sang to her.

My mother loved music, so I sang to her often. She was named after St. Cecilia, the patron saint of music, and for many years she was the church organist, as well as a gifted pianist and singer. One day, I was searching through several huge stacks of sheet music from the 1940's, trying to decide which song to sing. I chose one at random. Unfamiliar with the words and melody, I did my best to sing its sentimental love lyrics that held a bit of innocence, much like mother's youthful innocence at age 82.

While I held the music sheets in my hand, the musty smell of the yellowing pages filled me with memories of her sweet stories of old times. Singing, I sat on the edge of her bed, where she lay in her loose pink cotton nightgown with her eyes closed. Then suddenly, she opened her eyes as if wide awake and slowly turned her head towards me, her eyes shining with love and joy.

Although she was unable to speak, I could tell by the way her parched mouth opened ever so slightly that she had something to say, though the words would not come out. Instead, her thin, fading lips curled into a tiny, dimpled smile that made me imagine her as a schoolgirl again. She glowed with happiness as if remembering something dear to her, something that struck a deep chord. Then she lifted her left hand slowly and with great effort. Moment by moment, she wriggled her fingers deliberately, calling attention to her ring finger, with its loose-fitting silver wedding band still on. Her eyes shifted from her finger to me as her lips parted. There was something pressing she wanted to say, but it was a strain to speak.

In that moment, I realized what she was trying to say: it was her wedding song, the song she heard on the happiest day of her life.

My father was the great love of her life. Though he died of cancer seven years after their marriage, she never stopped loving him and never remarried. His presence was always a big part of our house, and his pictures were everywhere.

Each time I asked my mama if she wanted me to sing the song again, she nodded her head in affirmation. As the days passed, I sang that song over and over again.

Those days with my mother were extraordinarily beautiful and profound. They were also filled with much hardship and grief, especially after she had passed on, as I began to clear and empty the house. It was then that I grieved most of all, feeling the intense loneliness of knowing I would never see her again.

Yet there were moments when I felt her presence all around me, lifting, consoling, and reminding me that she was there and would always be there; only her form had changed. The love was there—it would not change or die, and it was within me.

She reminded me of something else too: the love, tenderness, and care that I gave her, I could give to other elders who, like her, were in the last days or years of their lives.

I remembered an old uncle from Poland whom Mama took care of until his death at 101 in the very same room where I took care of her. Affectionately, we called him "Fufu." I would sit with him, holding his hand while he spoke Polish to me. I never understood him and often asked Mama to tell me what he said, but she could not understand either. "His words are all mixed up and confused," she would say. "He doesn't make sense because he is senile and has something called hardening of the arteries." After he died, I told Mama I wanted to work with "old people." Three decades later, Mama reminded me of this calling.

Over the past eighteen years, I have worked in a variety of care settings with many different kinds of people from diverse socio-economic backgrounds. Some of the facilities were publicly funded; others were private institutions affiliated with different religious organizations — Episcopalian, Lutheran, and Jewish.

The work I do is about love — giving and receiving. The stories in this book portray the magic and healing that transpire through that exchange. They demonstrate the power of being present, listening deeply, and seeing beyond what appears on the surface. My hope is always to help restore a sense of wholeness and to facilitate the healing of the brokenness within each life I touch.

While this book focuses on the healing journeys of the elders, it also, without my intending it, touches on my own healing journey. It is about remembering dreams, mine and theirs, and even making some of those unrealized dreams come true. I hope these stories will bring inspiration, healing, peace, and well-being to the lives of your elders, as well as to your own lives. May you, too, see dreams come true.

1

NEVER TOO LATE TO LOVE

Essential points

- ◆ Aspire to be a channel for love.
- ◆ Bring love to all you do and observe its miraculous healing powers.

> *When doctors and patients understand the healing power of love, we will begin to add another dimension to medicine.*
>
> Dr. Bernie S. Siegel

Truly, love is restorative and life changing. Love can give life and return life even when it was supposed to have been taken away.

When Rodger came into skilled nursing, he had a brain tumor and was on hospice with three months to live. At 68, he was too young for skilled nursing. At first, his arrival kept getting postponed because he also suffered from obesity. The beds were not big enough, and we had to have one made that would fit him. It was no easy task.

When Rodger did come, everyone loved him, staff and residents alike, because of his sweet, good, nature. He could be gregarious and fun-spirited, though he also suffered from depression. It was as if there were something in Rodger bursting with life, but it was an incomplete life, crushed by the hardships he had endured.

The way Rodger's shoulders and head slumped over spoke of his inner defeat. *Was it his death sentence?* It seemed to me that that impending sentence may have been part of it, but there was something else too. He had not yet lived, really lived. He had never seen his dreams come true.

One day he shared with me how terribly lonely he was, saying that he had never married, although he always wanted to. "Maybe it was my weight," he confessed. "I don't know, but I've known plenty of broken heartedness in my life, when what I really would have liked is to have had one person to really love, who loved me too."

Maybe that was the deeper sadness I sensed. He also had no family. They all passed away, including his two older brothers who both died in a car crash not more than two years ago. He did, however, have lots of friends. His room was often filled with visitors, including staff, who also enjoyed Rodger's company. Yet as gregarious as Rodger was, the depression seemed to overcome him at times, robbing him of his self-esteem and confidence, keeping him from ever leaving his room.

Although the staff encouraged him to go to some of the programs, he always declined.

His supportive and encouraging friend Jim visited him every day and often spent hours at a time. Jim was always trying to persuade Rodger to get out of his room, even if for a short while, just to get some fresh air or to listen to music in the activity room. But Rodger rarely got out of bed. It was as if Rodger had given up on life, yet he still had not quite come to terms with his own death.

Then one Christmas Eve, Jim told Rodger how special the evening would be. A costumed choir would sing Christmas carols. Good food and wine would be served, with a choice of turkey with gravy, stuffing and corn bread, or fresh grilled salmon. Jim raved about the dining room's decorations of Christmas lights and a Christmas tree with lots of presents beneath–one for each resident.

Who could resist opening up a beautifully wrapped gift? Rodger also loved salmon, and although he had lost his appetite, he decided he would muster it up again for this one last Christmas Eve meal. With the help of several caregivers, he somehow found the strength to get up and go. He even combed his few thinning strands of hair and splashed on some aftershave. Dressed in a nice black jacket, and red bow tie, he was escorted in his wheelchair by his best friend to the dining room to a table set for four. Having arrived early, he told Jim he wanted to sit at a table close to the door, "Just in case if I get tired and want to leave early."

That evening changed Rodger's life. Shortly after his arrival, Billie Jo, a very pretty, petite lady was brought in a wheelchair by her private duty caregiver. As always, Billie Jo was nicely dressed. That night, she wore a pink chiffon lace dress and a red velvet ribbon in her short silver gray hair that had been curled and sprayed. Around her neck, she wore a pearl necklace and earrings to match. The moment Billie Jo saw Rodger, she pointed to him and his table. This was where she wanted to sit, she told her caregiver. At first, her caregiver did not pay any attention and kept wheeling her to the table she normally sat at, where all her girlfriends congregated, but Billie Jo got angry and, turning to her caregiver, insisted that she be taken *over there*.

"Where?" the caregiver asked.

"There," Billie Jo exclaimed impatiently, pointing to Rodger's table.

"Why do you want to go there?" the caregiver asked.

"I just want to sit with the nice young man. He seems like he needs company."

In that instant, Rodger turned to look at Billie Jo, who quickly transformed her nettled expression into a softer, more angelic gaze. With a coquettish smile, she batted her eyes. Rodger paused as if stunned that this pretty little lady was pointing and smiling flirtatiously in his direction. Then, in a sudden flash, his face lit up. He smiled, almost like a shy schoolboy, then waved his hand in a gesture of hello.

"Ah, I see," the caregiver said, and promptly took Billie Jo to Rodger's table.

At 4'11" and 95 pounds, Billie Jo was quite a contrast to Rodger, and at 93, she was 25 years older, still lovely and full of charm and warm heartedness. Unlike Rodger, who had struggled most of his life and worked hard as an insurance salesman, Billie Jo had never worked a day in her life. She had always been well-taken care of and pampered–and still was. Her hair was done twice a week. She had weekly manicures and pedicures, and was well-groomed every day. She had been married for 50 years, but when her husband had died 25 years earlier, she moved into the independent living section of this elder community until transitioning to skilled nursing when she was no longer able to care for herself. She never remarried and had spent all those years alone.

Like Rodger, she was lonely and had been for a long time. As lady-like as she could be, she could also be feisty and put up a fight if she didn't get her way. Had she not gotten her way about where to sit, she been prepared to battle with raised fists, to scream and kick, to wheel herself, if necessary, determined to get what she wanted.

On that magical, life-changing evening, Billie Jo had sparkles in her eyes and so did Rodger. All evening, she gazed at him adoringly, smiling and flirting coquettishly. Rodger enjoyed it immensely, and this was the first time I saw him look so happy. His face glowed, and his cheeks flushed as we staff glanced over from time to time, trying to be discreet, yet *oohing* and *aahing* and smiling among ourselves.

The following evening, Christmas day, Rodger and Billie Jo sat side by side over dinner. Their days of courting were beginning. They were together every evening, and every evening, they made special arrangements to have fresh flowers and a candle put on their table.

Rodger's depression became a thing of the past.

Valentine's Day came. They exchanged cards. He gave her chocolates and had a dozen red roses sent to her room. That evening, she dressed for the occasion, with red lipstick and a red silk dress and pretty scarf. He wore his red bow tie again, knowing how much she liked it because on Christmas Eve, she had complimented him on it.

Spring became their season, the season of blossoming love. Their caregivers took them for strolls in the park, where they could feed the wild geese and ducks by the lake.

Nothing could keep them apart, even though Billie Jo's room was the last one at the far end of the building and his was the first one at the other end. Quite a distance to travel on your own in a wheelchair, but somehow they managed, even when no caregivers were available to help them. Billie Jo would take herself in the wheelchair, moving with the speed and vigor of a tigress, as if her life depended on it.

Theirs was a song of love, with Rodger becoming a very different man. No longer were his shoulders slumped over. He held his head up confidently, and his eyes embraced a new vision: one that offered hope and healing. And healing rapidly he was. As the days and weeks passed, he did so well that he was taken off hospice. His three months turned into over a year. When I left this community, he was still alive and well, and they were still in love.

Further thoughts

Love goes beyond romantic love. Love is an energy that, when we're open, can come through us to bring deep peace and healing to the elders whose lives we touch. Love brings a sense of connection as well as joy, meaning, inspiration, and renewed life.

In *Love and Survival,* Dr. Dean Ornish writes:

> *Love and intimacy are among the most powerful factors in health and illness, even though these ideas are largely ignored by the medical profession... Love and intimacy are at the root of what makes us sick and what makes us well, what causes sadness and what brings happiness, what makes us suffer and what leads to healing. If a new drug had the same impact, virtually every doctor in the country would be recommending it for their patients ... When you feel loved, nurtured, cared for, supported, and intimate, you are much more likely to be happier and healthier. (p.3)*

Suggestions for creating engaging and inspiring activities

◆ Organize an event celebrating love and romance. Invite your elders to share their stories. Ask them to bring photos and/or any keepsake items reminiscent of their love life.

◆ Plan a special theme week of love and romance:

- Show old romantic movies with well-known actors and actresses that were popular in your elders' era.

- Bring in romantic art from books or slides that can be found in the library.

- Read love poetry, celebrate, and share! (see suggested reading for titles)

♦ Organize an event celebrating love in action as illustrated in people who have accomplished great things
through love, such as Mother Teresa or Mahatma
Gandhi. Invite your elders to discuss who they think
exemplifies love for them. It doesn't have to be someone famous. It can be an elder's mother or son, or even
a beloved animal.

PART II

REMEMBERING WHO WE ARE, REMEMBERING OUR DREAMS

IGNITING THE FLAME

Essential Points

- Celebrate your elders' accomplishments, talents, and dreams.
- Honor their wisdom.
- Keep a sense of community alive and thriving.
- Involve family, friends, neighbors, and other members of your community.

> *It is never too late to become what one might have become.*
>
> George Eliot

Ben had a dream that he shared with me. It sparked a desire within me to make that dream come true. *It's never too late*, I thought, *even at 91.*

One crisp, cool afternoon, while helping Ben with his wool scarf, sweater, and cap for our outdoor stroll, I noticed a painting of an old, bearded rabbi on the wall. Knowing that Ben had been working on this painting for months, I exclaimed, "You've finished! Bravo! It's beautiful!"

Lowering myself to his wheelchair, I hugged him and gave him a kiss on his rough, whiskery cheek. He smiled modestly, shrugging his broad shoulders, and asked, "Do you really like it?"

"It's exquisite. You've infused it with life. There's a soul inside that rabbi, who looks like at any moment he will turn around and speak."

Ben smiled, revealing the dimple in his right cheek, proud of what he had accomplished; yet there was a certain humbleness in how he tilted his head before saying, "Thank you. I put a lot of thought and time into it."

As I slipped the cap over his balding head, I noticed upon closer study that the penetrating blue eyes of the rabbi, with his bushy white brows, resembled Ben's, except Ben wore thick, wire-rimmed glasses. There was one other slight difference as well: a glowing fire inside the rabbi's eyes that held a prophetic vision. Ben's eyes also had that fire, except there was a sense of defeat, a certain loss of confidence that seemed to diffuse the flames.

As we went for our usual stroll, along a winding path strewn with autumn leaves, we continued talking about what we always talked about: art. Just five years ago, Ben, inspired by the elder community's art program and teacher, took up painting. It was his "new career," as he put it, and he pursued it in earnest. Each day was in some way devoted to his art. In a sense, it became a part of his religion and deep spiritual life. Often we talked about religion, but on that day, after two years of knowing Ben, I discovered something about him that I hadn't known before. When I commented on the resemblance between the rabbi's eyes and his, he shared with me how he once had a dream to become a rabbi.

"So, then the resemblance was intentional?" I asked.

"No, that was not my intention at all. I studied the portraits of rabbis and prophets. It came from what I saw in books." Yet there was a resemblance that could not be denied, and now I understood why.

"And why didn't you become a rabbi?" I asked.

"It was my father's decision, not mine. My brother was lucky. He got to do exactly what he wanted: become a rabbi. But I was younger, and when I was supposed to go to rabbinical school, the Depression came and everything changed. Times were hard. My father decided that it wasn't a suitable profession, so he decided I should do something more practical that would earn a good living, like become a doctor. So that is what I did."

In pursuit of his newly chosen profession, Ben abandoned his dream, but that dream never left him. Although he never formally became a rabbi, he was a rabbi in his own way: in his values and ethics, his forthrightness, his spiritual devotion, and the way he gave advice to others.

At the end of our stroll, we stopped in the garden outside the elder care community, a sprawling, newly-constructed complex set in the midst of rolling hills. I was working there as an activities therapist in the skilled nursing unit where Ben lived. There was also an Assisted Living section, as well as an Alzheimer's unit, separated by walls and doors that opened automatically with the right code.

Beneath ripening olive trees, we continued our conversation. I asked more questions and learned that Ben had helped found a temple, where he acted as a stand-in rabbi. While he was telling me about his past, I noticed a sort of wistfulness in him as he gazed into the distance at one of the highest hills, with an enormous tree perched on top. No matter what the season, he would often look at that lone tree. Its branches were leafless and jagged, resembling the hands and fingers of a wise old sage, pointing up to the heavens and beyond. That distant point reminded him of his unfulfilled lifelong dream.

Yet I saw how much that dream was still very much alive within him, its sparks never having gone out. It came out every day in almost everything he did, like in the painting of the old, bearded rabbi.

So I had an idea: to have a special program revolving around Ben as the rabbi. Residents, staff, family members, and friends would come to ask anything and everything they ever wanted to know about Judaism. They could also seek advice on how to live life. We would create a holy space where Ben could really live his dream.

With enthusiasm I turned to Ben and said, "Did you know … that *you* are *my rabbi?* I hope you know that, Ben." He raised his brows and looked at me in disbelief, as if to say, *I didn't think you were Jewish.*

"I may not be Jewish, but you are *my* rabbi anyway."

He smiled, then chuckled and asked me *why*, a question he asked often if I said or did something that intrigued him or made him curious, like one day when he asked why I do the work I do. After giving some thought to his question, I said, "It's work I have to do, Ben … I don't have a choice."

"That's a good answer," he replied. He responded like that often if he liked my response. Otherwise, he was silent or would nod his head or smile diplomatically.

After thinking about all the reasons why I would choose Ben as *my rabbi,* I said, "You are kind … wise… and knowledgeable, you are gifted, and because I like you best of all. You're the one for me." I was hoping for "That's a good answer," but instead he smiled and nodded. Then, without further thought, I told him about my idea and said we could call the program *Ask the Other Rabbi,* since we already had a rabbi at the community, and I did not want there to be any confusion. He liked the idea. I could tell by the twinkle in his eye, and the tone of his voice.

"All right," he exclaimed. Immediately, I called his daughter, Leah, to tell her about the idea. She was thrilled and knew that her father would be excited about it, too. The anticipated day of *Ask the Other Rabbi* became a day that Ben looked forward to. Something within him even seemed to change slightly. There was a certain lightness and cheerfulness, a certain confidence that seemed to grace each day. Soon afterwards, Leah and I had a meeting in which she shared some stories of her father's life. She also expressed her concern over her father's memory. "What if he forgets and doesn't know how to answer?" She was worried that it would make him feel bad.

I tried as best as I could to allay her fears. I wasn't worried about it, and apparently he wasn't, either. When Leah expressed her concern to him, he replied with his finger tapping the air, "Don't you worry! I'll have answers to give."

In the meantime, I told staff about the program, inviting them to come with questions. I also asked my husband, who is Jewish, for some questions. I really wanted to be prepared should there be any moments of uncomfortable silence. But when that day arrived, I did not have to worry at all. It was anything but silent. Or I should say, when there was a silence, it was profound, one that held more wisdom and wonder than words could ever convey.

Earlier in the day, I made it a point to show Ben the large white board on the wall with the listing of programs where *Ask the Other Rabbi* was featured prominently. He beamed happily. The normally drab dining room, which also served as an activity room, was brightened with fresh flowers and white table clothes. Ben's painting was displayed on one table at the front of the room. His bearded rabbi, whose eyes held the fire of a *prophetic vision*, was at the center, along with some photos of Ben's earlier life.

Ben and I stood outside in the hallway in front of the big, double door entrance that had been pushed open to accommodate the large crowd that had come to see him.

"Look at all the people waiting to see you, rabbi," I whispered.

With his mouth and eyes agape, he gazed around him, speechless. It was as if the spirit in the air had taken his breath away. He knew he had a mission to fulfill. The room was so full that a few residents were filing out the door and into the hallway. Dot, a feisty 95-year-old lady with wire rimmed glasses, tapped her cane furiously on the floor, demanding that she be brought to the front of the room. Sitting next to her was her friend Betty, a plump, good-humored 90-year-old woman, who kept telling her to relax.

"Everything will work out just fine," Betty whispered, while keeping her eyes on Ben, smiling and winking flirtatiously. She was hot for *this rabbi*. He knew it, and although he gave her a warm smile, he blushed and turned away quickly as I wheeled him through the expectant crowd. Nurses, caregivers, administrators, and social workers stood interspersed throughout the room. Among them were Filipinos, East Indians, African Americans, Nigerians, Ethiopians, Mexicans and Thais —a beautiful blending of accents, ages, colors, and nationalities there to hear the rabbi speak!

Leah, an attractive and articulate woman, stood waiting by the front table, beaming just like her father. She was pleased with the turnout and began the program by giving a lively introduction, which generated an instantaneous wave of enthusiasm and interest. In addition to telling us about her father's work as the stand-in rabbi at the temple he helped found in New Jersey, she also informed us about a meeting he once had with a well-known and beloved Jewish philosopher and mystic, Rabbi Abraham Joshua Herschel, who was a big inspiration to Ben.

As I held up one of the pictures of a tall, lean young man sitting down with a group of other musicians playing the cello, she proudly told us about Ben's brilliant side career as a cellist, a piece of his life that most of us did not know about. Although he could no longer play, it was still a big part of his life that came out in other ways, as in his paintings of cellists.

With his hands folded in his lap, and a big bright smile, Ben listened intently to his daughter. It was the first time I had seen him so vibrant, and happy. *Oohs* and *aahs* filled the room as I walked around to show his picture to each resident. The biggest *oohs* and *aahs* came from Betty and Dot!

Grabbing my hand holding the picture, Dot pulled it close to her face to have a better look. "I'll be darn!" she said. "What a handsome fella!"

Getting impatient, Betty pulled my hand in her direction, "Give it here, will you... Oh my! What a handsome fella is he, is right! Oh la, la, oh la, la, as they say in France. Oh la, la!"

"The juicy part is yet to come, ladies!" I whispered, taking the picture away to put back on the table, while Leah finished her introduction to a loud round of applause. Several hands waved in the air in gestures of *pick me, pick me, I have a question.*

I called on Juanita, one of the caregivers. In her heavily accented voice, she asked, "Can you explain what makes meat kosher?"

As Ben replied, there was a newly-found confidence and strength in his voice, as if he had not only had a gift for playing the cello and painting but also for speaking. "Animals were given life just as we were, and if we are going to kill them for our sustenance, it must be done in the most humane and painless way possible. A person called ..." Ben paused, while waving one of his hands in the air in a gesture of *what is it, what is the word I am looking for, as* Leah uttered the word, "shochet."

"... a shochet," Ben continued, "conducts this task quickly so that suffering is not prolonged. At the same time, he is blessing the animal, for its life is being taken away."

"Thank you," Juanita replied warmly.

A soft-spoken Filipina caregiver standing next to her asked, "Do Jews believe in an afterlife?"

"All rabbis speak of an afterlife, but there are many different views as to what that is," Ben explained, looking at his audience thoughtfully, taking in each person, as if wanting everyone to feel acknowledged. Lifting his index finger, he continued, "The mystics even speak of their belief in reincarnation."

"Reincarnation?" exclaimed Ann, a frail woman sitting in her wheelchair wearing her nightgown and slippers, her head and hands shaking uncontrollably.

"That's right, but only the mystics," he concluded.

"I see, because I never heard my rabbi talk about that," she retorted, bewildered.

"Only among the mystics," Ben reassured her.

Ben continued answering questions like a shining star. I was so proud of him. From time to time, I glanced over at Leah, and I could see she felt proud of her father, too. She was glowing. So was he. At one point, awed silence filled the room. At any moment, I felt as if that silence would burst with inspired whispers and heated talk about this Ben whom they had never seen before.

Breaking the silence, I asked, "What do you think is the most important element of Judaism, Rabbi Ben?"

Everyone waited in anticipation for his reply. "It is important for Jews to follow their chosen path, but to remember that it is not the only path. There are many paths, and it is important to remember and respect the many different ways. Truth is more important than religion."

I was struck not only by the beauty and wisdom of what he said, but also by his eyes: they glistened with vision. I glanced over at his painting of the rabbi. It was like a glowing shadow peering over his shoulder as his words poured out eloquently. Ben *was* that rabbi, and we saw an inspired soul who had been lying dormant for many years. As I looked around at the elders, I saw expressions of awe and hope.

I then asked Ben about his role as the stand-in rabbi at the temple he helped found, and the role that the rabbi should take in leading his congregants.

He raised his hands, as if his words were coming from somewhere beyond himself, and replied, "The rabbi's job is to support the spirit of the community, but it is important to not forget the individual. Sometimes a rabbi gets too caught up in the community at the detriment of the individual. Individual voices need to be valued and heard. It is important that each individual is not forgotten."

A sudden burst of applause filled the room. Ben paused to acknowledge the moment, as 98-year-old Miriam raised her arm with a clenched fist and roared, "Yes, that's right! Speak it out! We all want to be heard!"

Sitting in the wheelchair next to her was Bee. She shook her head in affirmation and exclaimed, "Yes, yes, yes!"

Jake, who sat with his legs propped up with tight bandages around his calves, shouted, "That's right! Our individual voices get drowned out and lost!"

Sylvia, who often dozed in her wheelchair during programs, suddenly opened her eyes and said, "We've got to do something about it!"

It was clear that the residents were no longer relating what Ben said just to the rabbi and his congregants. They had expanded it to other institutions because it struck a chord within them. They understood what every elder who comes into skilled nursing understands: how it feels when your voice is not heard and your confidence and dignity slip away. Ben was stirring them up and returning to them what they had lost. He was giving them back their voice and empowering them. He was doing his work – the work of the rabbi.

Everyone sitting in the room seemed to be transformed. I believe that even those elders who were not cognizant could feel something; maybe they could not define it or use words to describe it, but something powerful was happening to each person. Even Mary Grace, who normally slept during programs, lifted her head, opened her eyes wide and watched Ben intently. Although she was no longer able to speak, except for a few inarticulate words every now and then, her eyes followed each new voice that spoke.

There were no background whispering or talking, which was a rarity. There were no sounds of agitation, boredom, or discontent. A presence held sway in that room. Ben was being seen for who he was at his best, speaking his deepest truth from the most authentic part of himself. He had reclaimed what he had lost, what they had lost.

"You have a beautiful soul," Bee shouted while raising her arms in applause.

Other people chimed in with applause, as Miriam exclaimed, "Ben is a man of very few words but when he speaks, he has something very deep to say."

Before the program was over, I held up the painting for everyone to see and said what we all knew, "What a gifted human being we have here with us today. Let us give thanks."

Discreetly, I turned to Ben and gave him a wink, recalling that one autumn day when I looked at the painting and saw a soul within the canvass that I thought would at any moment turn around and speak.

More applause filled the room. When the program was finished, both elders and staff commented on what a wonderful event it was, and how they had no idea that Ben wanted to be a rabbi. No one had ever heard him speak so eloquently. No one knew that much about his life, and who he was as a person. He had touched a deep place inside of everyone, even Betty who was always the joker. When I asked her how she liked the program, she had tears welling up in her eyes. Shaking her head in amazement, she said, "He is really something else. I never knew he had all that in him. Amazing."

The wave of excitement and Ben's confidence continued even *after* the program. One of my colleagues commented on how assured he was in the singing group that week, a self-assurance that she had not seen in him in a long time.

Leah was very pleased and expressed her gratitude, saying how honored her father was on that day and how much joy it had given him.

And there was something else that was quite remarkable as well that I could not help but chuckle over: not once during the program did Ben cock his head and squint, pointing to his hearing aids with a look of bewilderment. This was his usual way of letting you know he could not hear. Leah called it selective hearing: if he *didn't want to hear* what you were saying, he would respond in this clever way. When he was bombarded with questions from social service, he used this technique quite effectively. But he was all ears on the day he lived his dream as "the Other Rabbi."

Further thoughts

When elders are put into an elder care setting, whether voluntarily or involuntarily, they may feel less valued, or think their ideas and opinions don't matter. Throughout their lives, they were here, in the center, but growing older, especially in a care setting, they find themselves suddenly cast out of the center, over there, on the outside. Helping our elders remember their accomplishments, as well as celebrating their lives, gives back their voice, with the message that they are important and valued.

It may even be possible in some small way to help an elder realize an unfulfilled dream. We see in Ben's story that this realization can empower, restore confidence, and give greater meaning to life. Creating a safe space where an elder can live that dream can be incredibly healing not only for the elder but for the entire community. Suddenly, waves of inspiration and hope reign as other elders begin remembering their dreams and feeling as if they too have something to say and are back to the center.

Suggestions for creating engaging and inspiring activities

♦ Ask your elders if they have an unfulfilled calling or dream. If possible, organize an event for an elder to actualize his or her unfulfilled calling or dream. For example, an elder may have once had a calling to be an actress. Is there a way of helping her perform a scene from a play, a soliloquy, or even the entire play, with other elders getting involved in the production?

♦ Or perhaps an elder has a lifelong wish to visit a foreign country. Create a day where that country is brought to him through pictures, music, dance, poetry, food, and/ or a travel documentary.

♦ Organize a sharing circle for your elders. Invite them to bring an object, picture, or story that tells of their dreams, both fulfilled and unfulfilled.

Some questions to consider asking your elders:

♦ Did you ever have a calling that was not fulfilled? Do you look back with a sense of regret? Why was this calling not fulfilled? What did you do instead? Did that give you a sense of purpose, or did you feel that something was missing from your life? What brings greater meaning into your life? What gives you a sense of purpose?

♦ If you could live life all over again, would you change anything?

♦ What were your dreams in childhood? Having a career? A family? Travel? Did you have any hobbies or games that you were passionate about? What kinds of things did you love to do most?

♦ What were your dreams in adolescence?

♦ What were you dreams in early adulthood? How did they change over time? Were these dreams fulfilled?

♦ What were your dreams in mid-life? For travel? For career? For family? For hobbies or interests? Have they been realized? How have they changed over time?

♦ What were your dreams at retirement? Are they being fulfilled in the present? Have they changed?

♦ Was there something or someone who inspired your dreams at any stage in your life? Who? What? When? Do you have any pictures, particular songs, or objects connected with your dream that you'd like to share with others?

♦ What hobbies and talents did you have but are no longer able to do? For example, painting, knitting, playing the piano or any other instrument, making jewelry, sewing, needlepoint, writing poetry, gardening. Is it possible for you to do any of these now in a limited or modified way?

♦ What hobbies or interests did you have that were never pursued? Do you still have those same interests, such as mastering a sport, musical instrument, or particular art form, like weaving, crocheting, quilting, or painting? Learning a new language? Volunteering for a cause you believe in?

SEEING WITH WHOLENESS

Essential Points

- ◆ Provide choices that encourage, invite, and support your elders.
- ◆ Don't let judgments taint your vision.
- ◆ See the best in your elders.
- ◆ Focus on what your elders can do, not on what they can't do.
- ◆ Create community. It has the potential to be a powerful source of healing, growth, and nurturance for your elders.

> *She has been with me all day,*
> *yet now it is as if I see her*
> *for the first time...*
> *She has been speaking to me all day*
> *yet now I finally hear her story.*

Mavis Muller

Sara had been at the community for nearly four months, yet I really did not know her as I did some of the other residents. She kept to herself most of the time, and I always got the sense that she did not want to be bothered, so our conversations were usually brief.

Sara had dementia. A former Professor of English Literature who had been known as quite the conversationalist, she was constantly frustrated by her inability to express herself as fully as she once could. If you asked her what kind of work she once did, or where she came from, words often got scrambled, or she would forget the word she was looking for. Flinging her arms into the air, she would make circular motions with her hands, as if to say, *what is it, what is that word, that idea, that profession, what is that place called where I was born?* When the word would not come, she would drop her head, pressing her hand to her forehead out of sheer exasperation and frustration.

Rarely did she come to activities, but she *did* come to Ben's program, *Ask the Other Rabbi,* and something marvelous unfolded within her. The expressions on her face began to change from discomfort, constriction, and pain to joy and openness. There was an aliveness gleaming in her eyes. She became so enthusiastic. Her hands moved around excitedly, as if she wanted to express how moved and inspired she felt about the program and Ben.

Often she spoke in fragments, and it was up to the listener to decipher the meaning, but it did not take long to understand Sara when she threw her arms up and exclaimed, "This is marvelous, this is so wonderful and marvelous. I had no idea. I had no idea."

"Yes," I replied, "I don't think any of us knew what a gifted and wise human being Ben is. He is beautiful, isn't he?"

"Yes, yes, yes," she said, clapping her hands, moving her tiny, frail body around in the wheelchair, as if she could not contain her excitement. It was already the end of the program, but Ben was still there. The room was still packed, with Ben glowing in his new roles as Rabbi, scholar, sage, gifted artist, eloquent speaker, and cellist. Ben had been recognized for who he was, not for who he appeared to be on the outside—an old man with hearing aids, sitting in a wheelchair.

One day after a dear friend and I had a deep and heartfelt conversation, I told her that I loved her. And she replied, "You love me because I see you." I could not help but to reflect on those words. Isn't that truly what we all really want? To be seen and heard for who we are, not who we are judged to be, or for what we are lacking, or what we are not and will never be, but for who we are in the truest, deepest essence of our being–our authentic self. Some people seem to bring out the best in us. We feel energized as we glow and shine in their eyes. They see us. Perhaps that was why the program *Ask the Other Rabbi* was so uplifting to Ben and to those who came.

After the crowd dispersed, Sara asked me to take her to her room, where she told me more about herself and showed me *her work*. She also was a painter, and her walls were covered with her paintings. A seascape, an impressionistic countryside scene, a little girl playing the violin, a ballet dancer, a still life of a vase filled with fresh flowers with petals falling to the table. Showing me her arthritic hands that had stiffened like claws, she expressed how sad she was because she was not able to paint anymore. It was too difficult to hold the brush, but all *this* was what she had once done. I knew what she was asking me, without directly asking the question: she wanted to have a day like Ben, where she could shine, *be seen*, be recognized and appreciated.

It did not take long for me to say, "Sara, your work is beautiful. I would like to do a program featuring your paintings. Would you like that?" Inspired by the art teacher at the elder community, I had started a program where resident artists were featured in a special program each month, similar to what I did with Ben in *Ask the Other Rabbi*.

"Oh my," she said, with her hand touching her heart. "It would be an honor for me. Oh my, oh my," she said sighing, still holding her hand to her heart. "Oh my," she repeated, beaming. "I would be delighted."

When I asked her questions about her paintings, I could see how she much she loved talking about her work. It made her feel proud and stirred something in her that she had lost, that many residents lose upon entering skilled nursing — the essential part of herself, with its many gifts and talents, having accomplished many things at an earlier time. On that day she began to remember... Although she saw her own work every day, she essentially had forgotten.

My relationship with Sara began from that day forward. I learned a lot from her and enjoyed getting to know her, although it required patience. My intention was always to try to understand, to listen, and to see the wholeness within the brokenness of her fragmented sentences and jumbled words. I began to feel what it was like to be in her shoes, with all its endless frustrations like losing the ability of full verbal expression, and having to depend on someone else for all your needs–like going to the bathroom, dressing and undressing, going to bed at night and getting up in the morning–when caregivers are too busy to take you when you want. It is never on your time, but on someone else's.

It was rewarding for me when I was able to understand Sara. And when I wasn't able to, I knew that simply listening was enough. Listening and being present are the greatest gifts that we can give to others. *Seeing* others for who they are.

Further thoughts

In Sara's story I wrongly assumed that her indifference came from wanting to keep to herself, but her indifference came from the activities staff not offering any activities that spoke to her. Inspired by Ben (chapter 2), she suddenly revealed her passion for painting.

Every elder has dreams, passions, interests, and accomplishments that often fall to the way side. Sara had stopped doing her art because of debilitating rheumatoid arthritis. Painting became a thing of the past, yet her love for painting was still there. That love did not diminish; it just required *remembering*. Although she could not paint again, she could have a show celebrating her work and could talk about it. It was her time to be *seen* and heard.

In discovering Sara's love of painting, I realized something important. My initial judgment of who she was got in the way of my really *seeing* her. We all have this longing to be seen for who we are at our best, as Ben was *seen* in his program. Ben's program ignited a spark in Sara, and that spark helped open my vision to other parts of her I'd never seen and may never have known.

Suggestions for creating engaging and inspiring activities

♦ Organize an event celebrating your elders' accomplishments. Focus on one individual at a time. Invite each elder to bring objects, stories, pictures, or anything else that illuminates his or her talents and/or accomplishments, those things that other elders in the community seldom have the opportunity to see. Send out invitations to family, friends, staff, and other resident elders. Create the space for each elder to bask in his or her light. Remember that accomplishments don't have to be big or grand. They come in all shapes and sizes.

Some questions to consider asking your elders:

♦ What kinds of films do you enjoy most? What are your all-time favorites?

♦ If you had three wishes, what would they be?

- What are you proud of?

- If you received an award, what would it be for?

- If you could do anything you wanted, what would it be?

- Who do most admire? Why?

- If you could go anywhere in the world, where would it be?

- Do you like animals? What kinds? What qualities do they have that you most like? Did you have pets? Would you like to have a pet now?

- What kinds of books do you enjoy reading?

- Are there any particular books that changed or shaped your life?

- What kinds of music did you listen to while growing up? Did your musical tastes change? How have they changed?

- What kinds of music enliven you? What kinds uplift your spirits or make you feel like dancing?

- What kinds of things make you smile and feel happy?

- What does the word "God" mean to you?

- What makes you feel most alive?

- What five adjectives describe you best?

- For other questions, please see chapter 2.

4

HER LAST PAINTING...
THE HEALING POWER OF ART

Essential Points

- ◆ Foster art and creativity.
- ◆ Explore old forgotten talents, and discover new talents.
- ◆ Create opportunities for your elders to feel "seen" and honored.

> *I dream my painting and then paint my dream.*
> Vincent Van Gogh

In my office above my desk, I had a painting of dots in different colors and shapes. Some were small, others bigger, some barely visible on the canvas, others squiggly, as if the hand had a hard time holding the brush still. They looked as if they had been placed on the canvas randomly, but something told me when I studied them closely that each dot had its own reason for being there and expressed the creator's intention. Each dot contained a few last wishes, held in relation, one to the other.

This painting was done by a 99-year-old woman who had not painted a day in her life. This was her first and last painting, and she had worked on it three times a week for a year. With a shaky hand, she diligently focused on those dots until she felt that she was finished. Not long afterwards, she passed away. To the outsider who has no idea of the story behind that painting, it didn't look like much, but to me it was beautiful because it held her story, her vision and dream.

I never met that woman, but each day I felt as if a part of her spirit were there with me. She had worked with a very gifted art teacher named, Eva, who started an art program at one of the elder communities where I worked. I remember meeting Eva briefly during my initial employment interview, and in an instant I knew that the work she was doing was important, and that no one else was doing it in quite the same way. In that instant I also knew that I had to work with her and see what she was doing. From her I could learn and grow. That marked the beginning of an inspired relationship.

Eva challenges elders and their notions of art and what that means.

Often someone will say, "But I am not an artist," or "I'm not creative. I can't do that." But Eva says, "We are all creative, and we all can create art."

Through art we can heal the wounds of our soul and of our past. What better time is there to do work on that deep level, than during those last years of our life – the time of preparation for the unknown journey ahead?

A day never passed when I did not feel awe for the work Eva was doing. Her students' paintings were displayed throughout the building. It was like going into an art gallery. The only difference was that many of these paintings were done by residents who had never painted before, yet these same paintings went out on a traveling art exhibit in museums throughout the San Francisco

Bay Area. Going into Eva's art room was like going into a temple. She had created a very special and sacred space, where silence was honored and where residents from both skilled nursing and assisted living worked side by side in the process of creation.

Inspired by Eva, I developed an on-going program in skilled nursing where each month a different resident artist would be celebrated through a special art reception. I hoped that by giving them this inspiring opportunity, it would not only make each of our residents feel honored and *seen*, but also it would provide an opportunity for staff and other residents to get to know their fellow neighbors on a much deeper level. My wish was that it would serve as an inspiration for all the residents and their family members.

My goals and hopes had been truly realized. I saw how much dignity and honor the program brought not only to the resident artists, but to every resident present. Eventually, the program expanded to include not just new artists but also residents like Sara who had once been artists. It also included other creative arts such as poetry, pottery or crocheted items. It kept expanding until it included nearly every resident. Not everyone chooses to paint, but everyone has a talent or skill of some sort that can be honored.

Further thoughts

We don't have to create a masterpiece. All we need to do is be open to whatever may come, without expectation. It is important to not focus on the end result, but rather to be present to the process of creating itself.

Many of us have a limiting notion of what creativity means. Remember that creativity comes in many forms—painting, sculpting, writing, singing, playing a musical instrument, arranging flowers, gardening, dancing, weaving, quilting, sewing, knitting, arranging a doll house, making hats or jewelry, etc.

But what does "being creative" mean? I once knew an elder who didn't think of himself as creative, yet at one time he loved walking by the sea and collecting pieces of driftwood that he carved into animals. He had a whole collection of driftwood carvings. I knew another man who collected musical instruments from around the world. That's creative too! Yet both thought of themselves as uncreative. Josephine had a talent for arranging flowers. Isn't that creative? And it's never too late to begin something new, or to resurrect an old passion.

The word "creative" can be daunting for many. When trying to encourage an elder who might be put off by the word create or art, try omitting those words from the invitation by saying: "Do you want to make something with me?" "Can you help me make this?" "Let's make something together." And before you know it, your elders are exercising their creativity boldly, brilliantly, and beautifully!

Even if your elders are unable to use their hands or their eyes, you can still explore what they've done in the past. Provide them the space to show their work to the community. Remind them of the beauty they once created.

Remember that it is never too late. I once worked with an 89-year old woman who took up the cello at 87 and practiced diligently every day! The process of bringing something to life is magical and transforming. It has the power to heal the brokenness within.

Suggestions for creating engaging and inspiring activities

Facilitate a group of elders to reflect on and discuss the following questions:

♦ What are your dreams, prayers, wishes, and hopes for the present and the future when you are gone? For your family? For your friends, both living and deceased? For the world?

♦ Invite them to write their thoughts down on a piece of paper or if they are unable to write, use a recorder. Ask if there are pictures, objects, or images that represent those hopes and dreams? If so, consider inviting them to make a collage. Or perhaps they might want to create a poem, a painting, a story or a song.

Three wonderful non-profit organizations that do art outreach programs with elders in long-term care communities are: Art With Elders in the San Francisco Bay Area; Elders Share the Arts in Brooklyn; and Art for the Aging in Maryland. They all use the arts to explore creativity. You will find their websites listed in the suggested reading and resource section.

I am most familiar with Art With Elders. Some of the elders I've worked with have had their paintings exhibited in their yearly art show and displayed at various museums throughout the San Francisco Bay Area.

The way these organizations work is different from 'art therapy.' Art therapy employs licensed psychotherapists, who may or may not be artists, to work with individuals in therapy sessions to address specific issues – depression, schizophrenia, anger, etc. In contrast, the three organizations mentioned above employ professional artists to oversee elders who simply want to learn to paint or draw. While the goals of art therapy and art exploration may be different, often the approaches reach the same place. I have seen miraculous transformations within elders once they begin creating their own paintings. This healing is a natural result of the creative process.

One elder with schizophrenia battled her whole life with issues of rage. For many years she was estranged from her son, but something remarkable happened during those last years when she began to paint: her schizophrenia not only seemed to dissolve, and so did her rage. As a result, her relationship with her son began to heal, and she died a good and peaceful death.

Suggestions for creating inspiring and engaging activities

◆ Bring in more creative arts. Start an art program, a theatre program (put on a play), or a drumming circle. Considering bringing in poetry and expressive writing, or dance therapy.

◆ Organize art shows where your elders can display their work. Remember art comes in many forms – it doesn't have to be limited to painting or drawing.

◆ Spotlight a particular art form each month, such as photography, dance, sculpture, weaving, knitting, and quilting. Show videos and slides of different artists and their work.

◆ Hold more poetry readings and storytelling events! In the suggested reading section, I've included titles of some books that elders have enjoyed immensely.

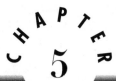

5

BEE'S WONDEROUS WORLD

Essential Points

♦ Turn the elder years into a time of blossoming.
♦ Discover new talents.
♦ Keep your elders thriving through creative engagement.
♦ Encourage your elders to bring beauty and joy into their living spaces.

Not I, not I, but the wind that blows through me.

D.H. Lawrence

"What is it that inspires you, Bee?"
"Spirit," she said.
"And what is spirit?"
"That which we cannot see."
"How long do you work on a painting?"

"It depends."

"What do you mean?"

"Only spirit knows. It's not up to me."

Bee and I sometimes had conversations like this. I liked to ask her questions to get to the heart of the matter of who she was, of what made her tick, how her mind worked. The conversations were never quite that smooth and easy. It took a lot of digging and much patience to understand Bee. She had lost her ability to speak in the way she once used to.

In spite of this limitation, Bee is an amazing woman. Her world is one of constant creation. She burns with a creative energy that is unceasing. In her small shared room with a single bed by the window, a room that initially had the typical sterility of most skilled nursing rooms, Bee has transformed her living space into a delightfully whimsical place of playful beauty. She has surrounded herself with all her creations — bright, lively paintings that adorn the walls, clay figurines of elephants and wild animals, clay bowls and wildly colorful papier mache animals.

Bee's work is unique. She almost never works from a picture, preferring to plunge into the depths of her own imagination. She loves painting with little dots. "There is a name for it," she would often say, forgetting what it is called. "Pointillism," I would remind her. Her work is never of landscapes or of people, but of shapes and designs, as if floating in space. One of my favorites is called *The Cosmic Egg*, painted in lavender with golds, yellows, and mauve. Truly, it looks just like its title, as if at any moment the universe will sprout from that egg.

Her work has been on display in elder art shows in museums across the country. But that is not where her creativity ends.

Bee makes jewelry as well. Strands of necklaces hang ornately from a hook in the wall. She has designed the large marble-size beads made of papier mache in vibrant shades of red, orange, purple, yellow, green. Some are painted with little dots, wave-like shapes or flower-like images. There are other necklaces as well, whose beads she did not create, but that she designed and strung herself. Dried out leaves, a rock or a shell sit by her night table to inspire her. Sometimes she forgets why they are there. Other times she remembers and will pick them up to ponder, studying the tiny veins in the leaf, or the way a rock feels at her finger tips with its tiny bumps and ridges.

She always carries a little notebook to write things down when she thinks of them. It doesn't have to be much, a word or two, a memory from childhood, a fragment of something, a word she saw in a book, or in a sign, something that holds meaning for her. This is Bee's world that she has created for herself during the last years of her life.

Bee never painted before taking Eva's class, nor did she do any of these other artistic endeavors. In many ways, Bee has made this time in her life one of growth and blossoming. I never think of Bee as having problems, yet I know she has plenty. She is confined to a wheelchair and relies on a caregiver for all things. She forgets words and how to string sentences together. I sit with Bee trying to get at what she wants so desperately to convey, until I slowly begin to understand. Then, I say what I think the word or words are, and when I get it right, she waves her hands in affirmation.

Seemingly out of nowhere, Bee will sometimes blurt out a word. One day the word was *enigma*. My assignment to her was to write whatever she could come up with about that word and what it meant to her. I knew it was significant in some way because she kept repeating it several times in one day while pulling out her notepad and pencil, as if in deep concentration over that word. Sometimes she would come up with other words, and we would try to decipher their meanings and string them together in a poem.

One day I brought in a box with dried-out autumn leaves and asked her to pick one that spoke to her and then, write a poem about it. She closed her eyes and let her hands skim over each one with a light touch, feeling for the right one. Picking one up, she opened up her saucer-like, penetrating eyes, studied the leaf closely through her reading glasses, and then shook her arms excitedly as if saying *this is it, this is the one.*

"What is it Bee?" I asked.

"Forest, a windy path, damp, wet, autumn…" Suddenly she paused, her eyes searching an invisible distance for the words. In her mind's eye she probably saw images or felt feelings, but the words themselves were lost.

"What is it?" I asked. "What color, what shape?"

Lifting her glasses, she kept searching, then blurted, "Hot leaves falling, sun, camp, children."

"Is it summer?" I asked.

"That's it. That's it!" she exclaimed, clapping her hands. "Summer camp in New York."

This was how we worked with one another, slowly whittling away until we discovered what was trying to come forth. Sometimes, she would get frustrated and want to stop, or I would ask her to write something for the following day. Sometimes she would forget what I had asked her to do. Other times, she would remember and more words would be scribbled, and we would continue working, or she would choose to set it aside and leave it unfinished.

Bee was very intuitive. One day, just before I was leaving for the day, I thought about how I needed to have an eye exam. I was trying to remember the name of the place I once went to, with relatively low prices and a nice selection of frames. I finally thought of it as I was walking out the door, and there was Bee, sitting outside my office. She looked up at me and said, "That's it, Site for Sore Eyes." That was the name I had been trying to remember!

Another evening, just as I was leaving, she lifted the book on Tibetan Buddhism she held in her lap, uttering its title to me. "Get this book," she said. I thumbed through it. It looked like a book I needed to read during that particular time in my life. I bought it, and in many ways, this life-changing book gave me answers to questions that had been rolling around in my mind.

Sometimes we exchanged words which on the surface seemed so simple, yet they took on another meaning in another context. Once Bee asked me to take her to her room, but our exchange soon transformed into *having walked this path many times before, in many places, in many lifetimes.* "In this lifetime I am here to serve you," I would say. We would laugh and joke about past and future lives, a concept we both believed in. We promised each other that we would meet again in the next lifetime, and that we would remember each other.

When I was no longer working at this elder community, I went back to visit after having been gone for nearly two months. Bee was in the dining room with her back towards me. I went up to her, threw my arms around her and whispered in her ear, "Do you remember me?"

She turned her head and exclaimed, "How could I forget you? I love you madly."

"And I love you just as madly, Bee."

I have found that when we see what is whole in someone, instead of what is lacking, when we see their light without judging and criticizing their flaws, they *can* and *will* shine. It is inevitable. I also believe that while labeling and diagnosing have their place, and are essential, they can also be limiting. People are then put in a box with a label. If you see only that, then the person gives you back just the box you have put them in.

A friend once told me about a social worker who never looked at the diagnosis before meeting the person. She wanted to be free of ideas or judgments. She wanted to see the person in his or her own true light.

Bee had been diagnosed with schizophrenia. Whenever she interacted with professionals who saw her in that light, she behaved in very strange ways. I never saw that side. I only heard about it. There is a power and a gift in seeing a person as whole. Bee had people in her life who saw her light, who supported her and who provided a safe and loving space to be that light, and she did amazing things.

Further thoughts

Creativity keeps us in touch with our deepest selves. When we lose that connection, life becomes meaningless.

Bee is the perfect example of someone who embodies the creative spirit. Never having painted a day in her life, she discovered in her last years that she had a gift. She created a life she would have never been able to have in her younger years because of life's *busyness*—raising children, keeping a household, and working two jobs.

Although most elders living in skilled nursing will have some physical, mental, or emotional limitation, sometimes it is still possible, as with Bee, to shift perspectives on what it means to grow old by seeing what is possible, instead of what is not.

Suggestions for creating engaging and inspiring activities

♦ **Make individual collages.** Provide plenty of old newspapers and magazines with colorful pictures and newspapers. Invite the elders to look through, choose, and cut out the images, words or phrases that most speak to them. You may need to assist with cutting, or can provide images, and words, that are already cut out. You can also use anything else that will adhere to poster board with glue, such as fabric, feathers, rhinestones, glitter, ribbons, appliques, small shells or stones, dried leaves or flower petals, and old greeting cards. Add textures by using pieces of old cloth. Exercise caution with small objects when some of your elders are prone to putting things in their mouths. Never use glue that is toxic.

♦ **Make a group collage.** This activity in not only fun, but builds community and friendships. Follow the same guidelines from above, except you might want to choose a theme such as "bringing more peace to the world," "the perfect world," "the world we want to leave behind for our children," "nature settings," "childhood memories," or any other theme that the elders might want to use. Or simply trust in the intuitive process of each elder without choosing a theme.

♦ **Design keepsake boxes** for small treasures, jewelry, or other objects that your elder chooses. Old wooden cigar boxes work well. Paint or draw on the boxes, and design with any of the following: beads, glitter, sequins, buttons, appliques, old photos, buttons, pieces of cloth that have a special memory or meaning (like a piece of fabric from a wedding dress), or whatever else strikes your elder's fancy!

♦ **Make stained glass windows**. There are some wonderful preformatted designs of cats, flowers, butterflies, gardens, etc., that are available at your local arts and crafts store or on amazon.com. They are fun to do and beautiful to look at. Encourage each elder to make one for his or her window!

♦ **Create mandalas.** A mandala is a Sanskrit word that means circle. Mandalas are an ancient symbol of the universe used for spiritual and ritual purposes most commonly in India and Tibet. Mandalas are used for healing, centering, and meditation. They are believed to instill a sense of unity and oneness. The elders can either use the preformatted mandalas or make their own by taking a blank sheet of white paper, making a circle with a plate in the center, and drawing in the circle. It is a wonderful activity for centering, relieving stress, easing anxiety, and inducing a state of peace and stillness. For preformatted mandalas, there are many to choose from. I've listed a few suggestions in the reading and resource section.

- **Make greeting, holiday, or birthday cards.** Have your elders draw, paint, or write messages on the cards. They can also use old photos, fabric, magazine pictures, ribbons, glitter, buttons, or anything else that will adhere with glue to poster board or card stock. There are many colors of paper to choose from at most arts and crafts stores.

A good way to open up the creative channel is this:

- **Draw, doodle, and play on magic paper.** Magic paper is available at any arts and craft store or on amazon.com and is truly magic. All you need are some good brushes and water. Dip the brush in water and paint. When the water evaporates, the image disappears. Great for relieving stress, and always takes away the pressure of having to get it right, or make it perfect.

SEEING THE LIGHT WITHIN

Essential points

- ◆ Celebrate the dreams and accomplishments of all your elders, including those who might be more mentally challenged.
- ◆ Search for the hidden gems within each elder.
- ◆ See the inner light.
- ◆ Don't give up, keep exploring, keep trying something new.
- ◆ Research each elder's history thoroughly; find out as much as you can about each one.
- ◆ Love unconditionally. The human spirit always recognizes love.

Unless I love something, it cannot reveal itself to me, and every revelation fills me with thankfulness, for I am made richer by it.

Rudolf Steiner

Fannie would sit in the hallway in her wheelchair with her chin to her chest, mouth open, saliva dribbling out onto her lap and cotton top, its crew neck always stretched out around the neck, as if it had outlived its wear. Her cotton pants were always a lighter shade than what they once were, having been laundered one too many times in the elder community's industrial machines. Her mass of curly white hair fell disheveled to her slumped-over shoulders while she was snoozing.

I adored Fannie and would bend down, throw my arms around her and kiss her again and again on the cheek. It was something I would not take the liberty of doing with everyone who was sleeping, but with Fannie, it was different. She didn't mind at all. In fact, she liked and welcomed it. It seemed to give her renewed zest. She would turn her head to me, throw her arms up with gusto, and start laughing and laughing, a roaring, hearty laugh that would then be interrupted by a coughing spell.

She once was a heavy smoker, and the cough never left her, nor did the raspy, robust quality in her voice. Waiting for her to stop, I would wipe her chin and mouth with a wet cloth. Then, I would hug and kiss her again and again, and say, "Why, Fannie, tell me why is it that I love you so?" And she would start laughing again, uttering some inarticulate words that I only wished I were able to understand.

One day she said something that surprised me. It wasn't so much that her words, themselves, surprised me; it was that I understood. Each word that she articulated came out clearly.

"I love you too," she said. It was a rare occasion, a moment I treasured.

Fannie had Alzheimer's. Whenever she spoke, everything came out jumbled, yet she liked to talk, as if she were sharing with me some of her deepest concerns and thoughts. Often I wondered what it was that was bubbling within her. What was she trying to express? Was it the stories of her previous life? Tales of her loves? Or how she once sang and danced?

Or was it of her problems now? Was she giving me wise advice, like that of a sage on how to live the good life, or perhaps expert advice on men and marriage? I would never know, yet I knew that something simmered inside her. Sometimes I would see her clenching her fists, as if she were nettled by something, while propelling herself down the hallway at high speed. She was a feisty one, who had declined considerably in the year that I worked at this community.

When I first met her, although still in a wheelchair and unable to communicate coherently, she was sometimes able to get out of her wheelchair, and dance with the assistance of someone — and could she ever dance! Throwing her arms up, she would shake her stuff, as if she were still a young, spring chicken. She was outspoken, as well. If she didn't like what the staff were asking her to do, she would wave her hands in a motion of *shoo, go away*. If they kept insisting, she would rally with clenched fists and wouldn't give up the fight until they relented.

That was the Fannie I first met. Over the year, she became weaker and stopped getting up to dance and started sleeping more, after suffering from a couple bouts of pneumonia. Her daughter, Rita, had started to give up on her. Rita used to come on a more regular basis and loved photographing her — and Fannie loved being photographed.

In her younger years, Fannie was quite the social butterfly, flamboyant and glamorous in her dress. She wore floppy felt hats, berets, silk and satin dresses, boas, scarves, and jewelry, anything that sparkled with elegance. Rita loved her, yet over the year had stopped coming as much, frustrated and saddened by Fannie's decline. Not knowing what to think of the situation, Rita became despondent. She believed that her mother had become a vegetable, with nothing left inside.

"She doesn't even recognize me anymore," Rita once said.

"I think she does," I replied. My words did not convince her, yet I wanted to show her that there was something more inside of her mother than she thought. After all, I heard Fannie say, *I love you.* I heard her laugh whole-heartedly while throwing her arms into the air. She wasn't a vegetable. I really did believe Fannie recognized her daughter.

Suddenly, something hit. It was one of those *ah ha, that's it* moments. The idea was this: to have a special event featuring Fannie, a celebration of her life with all her accomplishments as a dancer, showgirl, singer, feisty rabble rouser, who in her heyday was quite the women's libber. It would be a program honoring Fannie, and I would do whatever I could to help make it special for her.

The tables would be covered with gold satin cloth to display all her photographs. Fresh flowers, hors d' oeuvres on silver plat-ters, wine and sparkling cider would add to the festive air and the photos would not only be of her later years while in skilled nursing, but throughout her life. She should be dressed in her best clothes, something glamorous, something she did not wear so often, with a pretty scarf and hat, and she could have her nails and hair done. I would escort her, as if she were a queen, into the activity room that would be filled with those who had come to honor her: staff, fellow residents, and family members. Yes! That's it! I know she will respond, just like she did when she said, "I love you."

Without further thought, I phoned Rita and told her about the idea. At first she was reluctant, but I persisted, with the vision unceasingly glowing within. I was determined, just as Fannie must have been throughout her life. When Fannie had an idea to do something, she would not accept no for an answer. Instead I imagined a big YES propelling her, paving the way for whatever it was that she believed in and wanted.

In no time her daughter got excited by the idea. I asked if she would come in, so that I could interview her about Fannie's life "Bring lots of photographs and anything else about her," I said. My goal was to gather as much information as I could, so that the three of us could put together a beautiful program.

Diligently, I took notes. Fannie was born and raised in the Ukraine. In her early teenage years she boarded a ship with her family and immigrated to America, where they settled in New York City. Her dream was to be a singer and dancer, but her father was a stern man, who tended to favor the boys in the family. They were given an education. They were given musical lessons, and each boy learned to play an instrument, but with Fannie it was different. She was a girl, and girls were not as important as boys. Their duty was to get married and take care of the husband and family, not to get educated, so Fannie suffered. She saw the injustice in how women were treated and didn't like it. She rebelled against it and would not take no for an answer.

As she grew up, she plowed forward with her dream. Although she was not formally trained, she taught herself to sing and dance, and eventually made her way onto the stage, doing off-Broadway musicals.

Fannie came from a Catholic family, and when she decided to get married, her father was not too thrilled when he discovered that her fiancée was not only Jewish but poor. He owned a small business but never made much money. Against her father's wishes, she married him anyway. Fannie never converted. Neither was she a particularly religious woman, but she did enjoy going to the synagogue because it gave her the chance to be social, to gossip with the ladies, and the most important thing of all: to see what they were wearing while she wore her finest.

After a few short years her husband died, and Fannie was forced to raise two children on her own. In spite of the odds against her as a woman, she managed to find a job as a job counselor/recruiter. She did more than just match the unemployed workers with the right companies — she would cheer them on. She became like their life coach. Many men came into her office, hunched over, despondent, having lost confidence and a sense of their own worth from having been unemployed for so long.

"Sit up straight," she would tell them, "and remember who you are, the power within yourself. You have it! It's still there, and yes, you can do it. You will succeed. Whatever you want, you'll get. You are gifted and talented. Now go out there and get 'em!"

Fannie turned out to be one of the hottest, most sought after job counselor/recruiters. She was given many bonuses and was loved by her employer because *her boys* had the highest success rate in finding jobs! As I listened to Rita, I could not help smiling, imagining my dear Fannie as that feisty young woman with a big YES propelling her forward.

After the interview, I went over to talk with Fannie. She was snoozing in her room sitting in the wheelchair against the wall, with her chin pressed against her chest. I lowered my body to meet hers, and with my hand touching her knees gently, whispered her name. When she awoke, I told her about the program we were planning. I was not sure if she understood, but she listened, then chattered in her usual way.

I could not understand, but she patted my head in an endearing way. *Maybe she really did understand, after all*, I thought. I pointed to the painting on the wall of a young girl playing a violin and realized for the first time, after interviewing her daughter, that this painting was one Fannie had painted. A gifted artist, she had not painted for many years. I had seen this painting almost every day, yet never knew that Fannie was the artist. Her name was never signed to it, and if it had been, it had faded.

I told her how excited I was to discover so much about her, and while pointing to the painting, I said, "I never knew you were such a gifted artist as well. It's beautiful, really beautiful." She reached for my hands, and after a few moments began talking in her usual animated way. *Was it a response to what I had said about her painting?* I don't know, but she kept talking and talking, then let go of my hands, and gesticulated wildly; I knew something was simmering within her. Perhaps she knew something wonderful was about to happen.

When that day came, I asked her caregiver to dress her in her best outfit, with a hat, a scarf, and a little lipstick.

"It's your day, Fannie," I said, "You are the star," while pointing to the listings of programs for the day. I could sense she knew what was happening by the tender way she held my face, looking at me with eyes that expressed understanding and a wakeful clarity that I had not seen before. I was awestruck. My deepest hopes and wishes for her were becoming a reality.

The room was decorated, just as I had envisioned earlier, with 20 or so 8 x 10" pictures displayed on satin, cloth-covered tables. Hors d' oeuvres were brought out on silver platters, along with wine, sparkling apple cider, and fancy plastic glasses. Fresh flowers were set on tables. The room quickly became filled with residents and staff. I wheeled Fannie, our honored celebrity, in through the crowd. She looked just as beautiful as ever, sitting in the front of the room, where she remained throughout the program, along with her daughter and me.

After I introduced her, everyone applauded. Fannie savored it all. She knew exactly what was happening. A beautiful expression of joy and wonder came over her face. *How did all this happen, this memory of a once lived dream!* She was not groggy or sleepy but wide awake and the star. Drinking it in, relishing each clap, she nodded her head again and again in recognition.

With liveliness her daughter told stories of her mother's life as I held up the pictures. The air in the room was charged. Energized by the excitement, Rita spoke enthusiastically, enjoying the process of sharing her mother's life with everyone.

Fannie watched and listened intently to her daughter. When Rita noticed, she paused, clearly moved. Fannie, then, reached up for her daughter's hand and held it as she now took the stage. It was her turn. She had something to say and wanted everyone to hear it. Although it was hard to understand her, it was as if she were adding something to what her daughter was saying, as if to say *yes, yes, I remember that, wasn't that a grand time; hey, but don't forget this part of the story!*

Although Rita could not understand Fannie's words, she understood that her mother was not a vegetable. There was something more inside her, an undying light that was acknowledging this moment and saying *yes* to it. The Fannie she once knew was still there. You just had to seek her out. Fannie did recognize her daughter and she still had the capacity to love, to listen, to hear, to heal, to respond, and to feel deeply. Fannie was remembering.

Everyone was charmed and captivated by Fannie and by her daughter's stories. When the program neared its end, Rita took photographs of her mother, while I held up Fannie's painting.

Turning to Fannie, I said, "You are an amazing lady." She then reached out and hugged me. While looking at her eyes, I pressed my nose to her nose, and she laughed her hearty laugh.

Just when we thought the program was over, one of the residents who had known Fannie for a long time had something to say. She remembered Fannie from her heyday and told everyone about the shows where she saw Fannie dance. Winking, she said, "Boy, could she ever shake it. Show them, darling, show them what you can do!"

Fannie replied in her robust voice, still difficult to understand but it was clear that she was responding to her friend's request. Gesticulating with one hand, Fannie tapped it in the air again and again, as if to say, *yeh, you got that right, that's right, that's right indeed*. Fannie then threw both arms in the air, gave a little *cha cha cha*, with a wiggle and a flirtatious wink and bat of the eyes. The audience applauded and Fannie roared in laughter.

With tears in her eyes, Rita expressed how moved she was. She never knew that this *was possible*. "I still can't believe it," she said, shaking her head.

I thanked Fannie for sharing her remarkable life with us. Reaching out for her daughter's hand, she then took mine. Afterwards, Fannie touched the side of my face with her hand, and looking directly into my eyes, articulated something, that seemed heartfelt and deep. She then hugged me. I knew what she was trying to say: thank you.

"Oh Fannie," I said, "Why is it that I love you so, why is it that I love you so?" Throwing up her hands, she laughed again in her rip-roaring, robust way!

Further thoughts

No matter how mentally challenged an elder with dementia may seem to be, there is always a spark inside. As illustrated in Fannie's story, finding that spark brings life. Mine the hidden gems that may not be obvious, and they may come to surface with a little digging.

Every elder is unique. Search for his unique gifts, talents, and interests. What was special and meaningful to her in the past? What brought joy?

If you are a family caregiver and have access to his book shelves, comb through to see if there are any books that stand out as having been particularly meaningful, with passages high-lighted or with a dried flower pressed in its pages.

What about photos from the past? Or a particular painting or object that might have been special to her? Did he play a musical instrument and have a favorite song? What moved her deeply in the past? Don't dismiss her because it appears otherwise.

PART III

MUSINGS:
WHAT REALLY IS FORGETFULNESS?

JOSEPH AND RITA

Essential points

♦ Use touch more. Touch is vital to being alive.
♦ Be present and listen, though you may not understand.
♦ Provide a caring touch that lets an elder know you are present and listening.
♦ Be a source of support and comfort.

> *Love bears all things, believes all things, hopes all things, endures all things.*
>
> 1 Corinthians

She lay in bed curled up next to the steel rail. She was turned away from me, something unusual. Whenever I was with her, she sensed my presence because it was familiar. I could be her daughter, a friend, her sister, even her mother. One day, when she was especially affectionate with me, resting her head on my shoulder, and smiling brightly at me, I believed she thought I was her husband!

Among a host of other diagnoses, Rita had advanced Alzheimer's and was in her late 70's. My relationship began with her one day when I saw her in the hallway leaning over the arm of her wheelchair, her head and arms dangling helplessly in the most uncompromising position — a position that she got herself into often. It must have been terribly uncomfortable, yet Rita no longer had the ability to express her needs. She was unable to lift herself, so I called for assistance to help prop her up with a pillow. Then, I picked up her bulky, plaid slipper that was forever falling off. With her legs elevated on the wheelchair, one leg always managed to fall to the side, with the slipper constantly falling to the floor.

I have a tender spot for fallen slippers because I know how difficult such a simple task as picking up a slipper can be for someone in a wheelchair. I've picked up many slippers, and Rita's was one. With great care, I handled it, slipping it on her foot.

I stroked her forehead and held her hand, something that I did often, while chatting with her, asking about her day, telling her about mine. Magically she would turn towards me, suddenly becoming animated. She liked to talk and would go on and on. I could not understand a single word, yet she spoke as if I understood, and as if she had much to say, catching up on old times.

She did not say much that day, as the late afternoon light of winter came in through the half-open blinds, leaving striated shapes across the white comforter that her husband had bought for her, with her name sewn in large red letters, RITA.

I held her hand, but it was cold, lifeless. Rita was put on hospice for the fourth time and had been battling pneumonia for several weeks. She was a tenacious one who always bounced back and was not ready to let go, but this time I feared we would lose her.

Yet why should I fear? If it is her time to go, *let her go and let her go in peace, don't hold on...* I knew that to be true, yet I adored her ... maybe because she reminded me of the grandmother I never knew.

I walked over to the other side of the bed and reached out to gently stroke her face. Her cheeks were sunken. That was nothing new because she never wore her dentures, but this time she had lost a lot of weight, and it showed in her emaciated face and torso. Always thin, she had become skeletal. She was not eating and hadn't been for quite a while. That was rare for Rita because she loved to eat, in spite of not having teeth. It did not matter what form her food took – mashed, blended, pureed or on the rare occasion, whole – she ate whatever was put in front of her. Now that is a sign of someone determined to keep living, but this time she no longer wanted to eat, not even a sweet, one of her real weaknesses. She looked as if death had already claimed her, and at any moment she would be whisked away in one last gurgling breath.

There was heaviness in her breathing. I could feel the fullness of her lungs and a strange sense of drowning came over me. I wondered: *What is she experiencing? Does she feel pain or has the morphine taken it all away? Can I do something for her?*

I gently pressed my finger to her skin, which was as fragile and thin as onion paper. I had studied acupressure and knew that certain points on the body can help with congestion. So I worked with the lung meridian, pressing and holding, then releasing, while sending silent thoughts of healing and peace. Minutes passed... Nothing.

The light shifted and began to fade. The days were shorter. It was December, the time of year when most deaths occur in skilled nursing. Often it happens in waves of three or seven. We had lost two already. Would Rita be the next?

I wondered, *what it is about winter? Is it because of the cold? Is it because of a dark loneliness that sets in, with the sun departing sooner? Or is it because we are connected to the earth, to the flow of the seasons, and winter is the time of letting go, a time of emptying out, when the fields are made fallow, so seeds can be planted in fertile soil for the spring germination? Or is it because visits dwindle? Does love suddenly feel absent?*

Rita certainly was not lacking for love. Her husband adored her. She was his *one and only* queen. I wondered if that could be part of the reason she persisted in her fight to live. Love is powerful. It transforms, sustains, and heals.

I have always been touched to see how devoted he was to her, in spite of the fact that she had become what some people would call a vegetable. Unfortunately, not all husbands are so loving. I once worked with a woman whose husband ran off with another woman and completely abandoned his wife, without visiting her even once. But Rita's husband, Joseph, came daily, morning, noon and night. In the morning he arrived with a copy of the *New York Times*, wearing his winter jacket and scarf, regardless of the weather and the season. He was always cold, even on a hot summer day.

Sitting by her side, he would speak lovingly to her, stroking her forehead and the side of her face. *What can I do for you, my darling? Are you happy? Did you get a good night sleep? Are they treating you well here, dear?* He would not go to lunch in assisted living until he made sure that she was fed, but he would have to wait, because she was not fed until the second feeding.

"It's O.K., Joseph," I would say to him. "Go have your lunch. You need to eat, too. I will take good care of your wife and make sure she is fed. So please don't worry."

After lunch he would return to see to it that her caregiver put her to bed. He knew she got sleepy and liked a nap. Always particular about who Rita's caregiver was, he wanted to make sure that she was kind, gentle, and caring. If he thought she was the least bit rough, he would request another.

"*You* are a model husband." I would say to him. "Every woman wishes that when she grows old, her husband will be just like you!"

"But, she's my wife," he would respond matter-of-factly with a boyish smile that said *golly gee whiz, you are flattering me,* yet he was always humble and steadfast in his idea that, *isn't this what we are all supposed to do?* Now that Rita was on hospice, he came even more often.

I pressed Rita's arm and held two more acupressure points, as I directed more thoughts of healing and peace to her – to her lungs, her heart, body and spirit. But *this time* something marvelous happened: I *did* get a response. Her breath came out in a long sigh, and she opened her eyes wide for one brief magical moment ... and mumbled something... Although I could not understand her words, the tone was sweet and endearing. *Was she dreaming? Did she think I was Joseph?*

Closing her eyes, she fell back asleep. *Will she wake up again? Will she bounce back to life again?*

When Joseph arrived, I left them to be alone with one another. While I was walking down the long florescent-lit hallway, with its spotted carpet, aware of how empty the hallway was — most of the residents were in their room or in the dining room having dinner — I began to remember my relationship with Rita and Joseph as it evolved over time. I thought about her life and his, or at least the little I had gleaned over the two years I had been there. He was proud of his wife. "She was a brilliant woman," he would say with admiration. "She was a scientist and a professor."

So was he. Together they had traveled the world. She loved gardens and gardening. Both were fond of animals, especially cats. That was something that we all had in common: cats, gardens, and travel. These were the subjects of our conversations, which would often repeat. Joseph was becoming forgetful.

I liked to remind Rita of all the amazing things I heard from her husband. "He is so proud of you, Rita! He told me what a world traveler you are. So am I! I've been to India four times! I've heard you've been to Africa, India, China, Nepal, Europe, and South America! That's wonderful, Rita. And you are wonderful!"

Sometimes Rita even replied, with a *certainly, good,* and *oh yes, oh yes,* while smiling and nodding her head. She seemed to be saying, *yes I do, I do indeed, understand,* her arms folded over her chest, with her head cocked as if in deep contemplation, something she must have once done often.

How much did she really understand? I will never know. Maybe it was more a feeling that she had, or memories restored like a series of fragmented, jumbled-up snapshots of other times, other places once visited. Lush and beautiful scenes, but like a jigsaw puzzle whose pieces lie scattered on a table. I have often wondered how her mind worked, how she saw the world and how memories appeared in her mind, but one thing was clear and certain: I heard her say *certainly*, *oh yes*, and *good*.

One day while listening deeply to Rita as she chattered away, Joseph stared in amazement. He thought that somehow I understood her, that I was some kind of miracle worker, who could decipher this new, enigmatic language that she spoke.

Furrowing his brow, he looked at me, stunned, and exclaimed, "You mean you can understand? My god! What does she say? I never understand a word she says. What's the secret?"

Laughing, I replied, "I have no secret. I too do not understand, and I do exactly what you do. Listen and respond. Listen and respond while showering her with affection." And that *was exactly* what he did! Although he could not understand her, it didn't matter. She understood something on an even deeper level, that he loved her.

On their wedding anniversary, he brought her flowers and a card that he wrote himself. While holding her hand, he read it to her adoringly, discerning the words through his oversized bifocals. He seemed especially happy on that day, smiling like I had never seen him smile before, as if that smile would whisk them both away to their honeymoon suite in the savannahs of Africa. He glowed as if falling in love with her all over again, like he did over 50 years ago. That was the same day that Rita gave me a big smile, with amorous twinkles in her eyes, right after he left for lunch.

I remember, too, her long-haired gray cat, whose 8 x 10 framed picture sat on a chest in her room. Her name was George, named after the 19th century feminist writer George Sand. I would take the picture and show it to Rita, while talking about her cat, George.

"What an adorable little feline George is. Cats are such great companions aren't they? You must love her... It's funny how they sit on your books when you're reading. Isn't it, Rita? I bet George sat on your books all the time," I said to her. Some days, she would touch the picture smiling, as if deeply connected to that image in the moment, while making unintelligible utterances as if she were trying to communicate something that only she could understand. Other times, she would gaze far off into space, as if she were not even aware of my presence, and not able to see the photo of the cat she once loved, there in front of her. She seemed lost in another world, one all her own. I could never predict how she would respond.

Her son, who came every once in a while, was taking care of their cat. Also a great cat lover, Steve, like me, tried persuading the administrator of the community to adopt a few pets. I had worked in another community that had a docile cat and dog, and I saw how they worked wonders for the elders. All communities should have animals, even if just birds in an aviary or fish in an aquarium. It is amazing how soothing it can be to simply watch colorful fish swimming in their natural splendor.

"Health regulations," was the reason I was told by the administrator.

"But it would be wonderful for our elders!" I replied.

"And who will clean up after them?"

"Our elders ... and if they forget, the staff. Somehow it worked in another community that I worked in." My petitions, like Steve's, went unheeded.

I settled for the next best alternative: asking if we could bring the cat in for Rita just for an hour or two. That was welcomed wholeheartedly as long as Steve had the paperwork for all George's shots.

Whenever I saw Steve, which wasn't that often, I would ask, "Did you bring George?"

"Not yet, but I will," he would say.

Later I found out that Steve had a troubled relationship with Rita and Joseph. I wondered if that was why he came in so infrequently and kept forgetting to bring George.

When I didn't see Steve for a while, I asked Joseph whether his son had brought George in yet. A confused expression came over him, followed by an anxious pause, as he replied, "George? Who's George?"

"Your beautiful kitty," I exclaimed. He still looked bewildered. "Look, I will show you," I held the picture up for him.

Smiling and reassured, he replied, "Ah! Of course, George! For a minute there, I forgot that we ever had a cat!"

As time passed, Joseph became more and more forgetful. Sometimes he would stop in the middle of the hallway and scratch his head with a look of bewilderment.

If he saw me, he would call me over and whisper, "Listen, I feel so embarrassed. I don't know what has come over me, but I don't know where I am, and I don't know where I am supposed to be."

"It's O.K. Joseph. There is no need to feel embarrassed, Joseph; we all get forgetful sometimes. We all lose our direction. Right now you are in skilled nursing, where your wife is. And you live in assisted living." Walking with him, I would point the way. Eventually, he was moved into skilled nursing into the same room with his beloved wife.

We really thought we would lose Rita this time, but for the fifth time, she was taken off hospice. And once again she ate voraciously, smacking her lips, a tenacious, rambunctious lady is she!

As forgetful as Joseph became, he never forgot his love for his wife. He still cared for her in the same way, always making sure that she was comfortable, that she had her nap in the afternoons, and was fed on time. Almost every day, he would ask where his room was.

"I will show you, Joseph."

Once we arrived, he would stand looking perplexed, thinking this was not their room. There must be some kind of mistake.

"Are you sure?" he would ask. Perhaps he wasn't quite used to his move from assisted living into skilled nursing. It can be confusing.

"I am sure, Joseph. Look, here is your name with Rita's. And if you look inside, you'll find all your beautiful things." The room was decorated nicely, with paintings they had picked up from their world travels, a tall wooden statue of a giraffe from Africa, pieces of pottery and vases, along with a display of nicely framed pictures of their grandchildren, and of course the cat.

There were also two dining rooms in skilled nursing, which made it even more confusing for Joseph. One was for residents who are more independent and can feed themselves. The other was for residents who require more assistance. Rita ate in one, while Joseph ate in the other. He could not understand why, and as he sat down at his dining room table after being escorted there, a frantic look always came over him, of *why is this happening, why am I here, and why is she there, why are we being separated?* Whenever I saw that expression, I knew that he needed to be reassured. He needed to have someone explain why they were eating in separate dining rooms.

Nearly every day I had the same conversation, as he very indignantly would ask, "Why am I here? Where is Rita, and why is she not eating with me?"

"Rita eats in another dining room because she needs more assistance than you do."

"But is she alright? Does she know where I am? She probably doesn't even know. Can you please tell her and explain why she is eating there and I'm here? And can you tell her that I will come back, to not worry, she won't be left alone."

"I will be sure to tell her right now, Joseph, without delay, so don't worry. And I will make sure she knows you will be back soon." That was enough to reassure him. He was then able to eat and converse peacefully with the others.

I did as he requested, although I knew that he was more worried than she, and that she probably had other things passing through her mind, like *don't feed me so fast*, since I once saw a caregiver spoon-feeding her all too quickly, shoveling food against Rita's mouth, which Rita had forced shut, not wanting to open it until she was allowed to swallow the last bite. I understood why Joseph was so concerned. When elders are not able to fend for themselves, things like that can happen more frequently.

I have continually been touched by the love that has sustained this beautiful couple. We all want to be loved, and most of us wouldn't want to be left alone and lonely in those latter years. Rita and Joseph were blessed. They had each other. Love was theirs, and isn't that a gift?

CHAPTER 8

WHO IS THIS I, ANYWAY?

Essential points

◆ Take time to reflect on this: "Who am I?".
◆ Take time to reflect on your how your identity is connected to and influenced by your work and your relationships with others.

> *Hidden in the heart of every creature*
> *Exists the [Divine] Self, subtler than the subtlest,*
> *Greater than the greatest ...*
> *Formless in the midst of forms, changeless*
> *In the midst of change.*
>
> The Upanishads

I am a writer, an elder care worker, a massage therapist, and a wife, but who and what lies behind *the I* associated with these names that have become a part of my identity? If my memory were wiped away, what would be left? *The I* that I thought myself to be would suddenly be snuffed out. How would I understand myself then? What would 1 think? What would the world look like? What would it feel like? Is that state like a place of limbo, a transitional space in preparation for leaving this life and going to the next, wherever that may be? What is it like?

I have read that in persons with Alzheimer's the regions of the brain connected with memory, mood and location become clogged with deformed proteins. Thus, over time, memory is slowly wiped away. Words become sparser, jumbled up and lost, until one's identity is forgotten.

The Irish-born philosopher and prolific writer Iris Murdoch was diagnosed with Alzheimer's at the age of 76. During that time, she was working on her last novel, *Jackson's Dilemma*. The critics were all disappointed when it came out, because it was completely different from anything she had ever written, but it wasn't the subject matter that disappointed them, it was her use of language that was so different from her previous writings. Not only did her vocabulary shrink, but her sentence structure was no longer as complex, nor was she as articulate. During the time she was writing *Jackson's Dilemma*, she knew something was just not right. Something was changing. She thought it was writer's block.

I imagine that most people in the early stages of Alzheimer's have that sense that something is just not right. I will never forget Gertrude, an elder I worked with in the beginning of my career. I had become quite fond of her and would massage her hands or take her in her wheelchair out for a stroll. I knew she had been diagnosed with Alzheimer's and was still in the early stages.

She always recognized me and had great affection for me, but she began to forget many other things, like words. She would be telling me a story and in the middle of a sentence would suddenly go blank and forget the word or words that came next. Then she would completely lose her train of thought and start talking about something altogether different. There was always a look of embarrassment, of not wanting to show that she knew something was wrong. She would also forget where something was, why or how she got there, or where she lived, or where her daughter lived.

One evening, as I was leaving for the day, I went into the dining room, where the residents ate together at one long table. I remember the chatter and rattle of soup spoons in half empty bowls in an otherwise silenced room. I went around saying "see you tomorrow" as I always did, but when I got to Gertrude to give her a hug and kiss, something she always looked forward to, she turned to me with an especially worried expression, while grabbing my wrist with an urgency I had not seen before. With tears in her eyes and choked voice, she whispered frantically, "I don't know how to say this, but something is wrong with me. I don't know what it is. Something is happening. I wish I knew what it was. I am not the same person I once was, and I don't know who I am anymore."

Another elder I served never expressed fear or worry over her condition. Instead, she clung tenaciously to her identity, always reminding herself and others of what she once did. She refused to let it go. Her name was Shirley.

Two to three days a week, Shirley sat outside my office in her wheelchair, her eyes revealing a certain recognition while she pointed at the sign "SOCIAL WORKER/ACTIVITIES." This was her way of letting me know that she was once a social worker.

Her daughter told me that as a child her mother's dream was to bring more peace, justice, and kindness into the world. Following that dream, it became not only her work, but her passionate calling – helping those, whose voices are unheard and powerless, those in need. Yet, not once have I heard her say the word, "social worker," although I did hear her say "skilled nursing." Each time we passed the sign in front of the double doors that magically open, she liked to stop, point to the sign and read aloud: "SKILLED NURSING." She seemed so pleased and proud that she was able to say those words.

Shirley had a form of advanced dementia, and her language skills suffered greatly. Rarely did she speak, yet she communicated her moods and needs in other ways.

I called her my angel because she reminded me of one with her white, silky hair and clear skin, and the glow within her blue eyes, radiating an angelic loveliness. Sometimes spotting me from far down the hall, she would run with her wheelchair to come greet me, lifting her arms, lips puckered, ready to kiss me. When I bent down to her wheelchair to give her a hug and a kiss, she would take hold of my face, shake her head back and forth, smiling, as if expressing *I can't believe it, this is too good to be true.*

She may not have had the words, but I understood her love and affection, and so I exclaimed, "You're just like an angel. Just like a beautiful angel!" Her eyes continued sparkling with joy.

Shirley wanted her daughters to be strong and intelligent, not afraid to develop their minds. She was an ideal role model, who stressed the importance of strength and independence, instead of weakness and dependence as women were often taught during that time. It was all right to be smart, she would tell them. Women did not have to less intelligent than men. She taught them not to fear, and to keep growing and learning.

"Your daughter Martha has told me so much about you!" I said to her one day. Martha once showed me a card with a two page letter that she had written for her mother with all the reasons why her daughters loved her. I liked to remind Shirley of that card and those words, of how beloved she was, and how all her daughters appreciated the way their mother had raised them.

Shirley always listened, nodding her head from time to time, her hands folded in her lap, smiling with a sweetness that seemed otherworldly. In those moments, I knew she was happy.

When she was not happy, she would let you know that, too. I've seen her angry, wearing an indignant expression, as if some great injustice had been done to her, arms folded over her chest, head turned away. She could hold on to that mood for hours. Other times, it would dispel quickly.

Shirley was transparent, always letting us know what was going on, although not in words. It was especially during these times that I wished I knew exactly what was bothering her. Was it something that happened in the present moment? Did I do something? Was it some unresolved conflict from the past that came back to her time and time again? Or was she angry with one of her daughters or son for something not said, not done, or done, but not in the right way? Martha once told me that her mother held high expectations for her children.

It was as if during those bouts of anger, that part of Shirley, the social worker speaking on behalf of silenced voices, was still there, except this time it was her own voice that she was speaking out for, and she would not let that voice be diminished. If she was angry, certainly, it was because something that was unjust or unfair. She would not give up, nor let us forget, always reminding us, through nonverbal expressions, and by pointing to the sign in big block letters, "SOCIAL WORKER," in her happy moments and angry ones, and anything in between. It was such a big part of her. It was what sustained her. It was how she knew herself for a good part of her life. Without it, where would she be? Who would she be?

IS FORGETFULNESS
REALLY ABOUT REMEMBERING?
(THE DIVINE SELF)

Essential point

♦ Reflect on this: Who would you be without your
memory?

> *Our birth is but a sleep and a forgetting:*
> *The soul that rises with us, our life's Star,*
> *Hath had elsewhere its setting,*
> *And cometh from afar.*
>
> William Wordsworth

The thought of growing old is frightening for many — the
thought of *forgetfulness* or of becoming *senile*, as my mother
used to call it, referring to my centenarian uncle who lived with
us until the time of his death at 104. When I asked her why his
words came out scrambled, or why when in the middle of telling

me a story, he would suddenly stop and stare vacantly into the distance — she replied, *Oh, he is just old and senile.*

At that time, the word *senile* did not have quite the same pejorative meaning. It was simply a way of describing the conditions associated with aging, such as *forgetfulness.*

Now we have other words in use that are more specific to the condition, such as *dementia,* a term used to describe the cognitive impairment associated with any number of disorders, such as Alzheimer's, brain damage due to a head injury or a stroke, and Parkinson's disease. Forgetfulness is a part of dementia, but it is not to be confused with the kind of forgetfulness associated with the normal process of aging.

When I forget something, like when I misplace my glasses or car keys one too many times in a week, or when I forget a word, or someone's name that was once so familiar to me, suddenly I am aware of the aging process. The forgetfulness associated with dementia such as Alzheimer's is progressive, and is caused by deformed proteins that slowly invade that part of the brain associated with memory. Over time, more and more memory is wiped away.

What a difficult process that is for anyone to digest and accept, yet perhaps there is another way to look at it: maybe it is about preparing for the bigger journey, the one that begins when this one ends. I am still relatively young. I still have many more years left before I retire. I am still in the late summer of my life, yet I know that years are advancing all too quickly, and eventually autumn will come, followed by winter, and the winter is the season for emptying, upturning the earth, making it fallow in preparation for the spring planting and harvest. Maybe it is time to surrender to the process instead of fighting it.

I don't mean that we should not do what we can to keep our minds as sharp, vital, and alive as possible. What can be done to strengthen our memories and sharpen our minds, should be done. What can be improved or changed should be, but some things cannot be changed, and maybe it is better not to fight, but to accept what is, and to surrender to life and where it takes us, wherever that may be, although we may not like it. One thing is certain: each day we are growing older and someday we will die.

Perhaps forgetfulness allows us to begin the process of letting go, letting go of our attachments to who we are, or at least, who we think we are in this body. And perhaps forgetting is really about *remembering who we really are* beneath the outer garment of this body — this garment that becomes worn, and faded, and eventually must be discarded. Perhaps the forgetting is really about remembering something bigger, something we have forgotten.

There is a story from India that is one of my favorites because it always gives me a glimpse into another way of perceiving, and one that reveals a certain depth of truth that may be hidden from us.

*It is the story of an ascetic, Narada, and one of the gods, Vishnu. According to myth, Vishnu has a dream. That dream is the universe as we know it, and one day Vishnu says to Narada, "I will grant you one wish." After giving it some thought, Narada asks to be shown the secret of Maya. ***

"Come with me," Vishnu says, as they walk together for thousands of miles across India, until they reach the hot desert sands of Rajasthan, when Vishnu says, "I am thirsty. There is an oasis nearby. Go and fetch me some water."

Narada did as he was told and found the oasis set in a lovely village of green fields. Wanting to first get permission for drawing the water, he knocked on the door of the first hut he saw. A beautiful young woman answered. The moment he set his eyes on her, he forgot his mission. Not only did he forget the reason he was there, but he forgot everything, except his desire for the maiden. They got married, had two children, lived a good life and were happy, but after some years had passed, an unusually fierce monsoon came. It rained day and night continuously until the entire village was under water, and their hut collapsed. Narada tried with all his might to hold onto his children and wife, but he couldn't any longer.

The water was too powerful, and they separated one from another, until Narada woke up face down on blazing hot grains of sand in the desert. When he opened his eyes, he saw Vishnu before him asking, "Where is the water you promised me? A half hour has already passed." Narada looked into Vishnu's eyes not knowing what to say. Vishnu then asked, "Now do you understand the secret of my Maya?

* Maya refers to the fact that we are often tricked or deceived by the world, appearances and life.

HIS IS A SECRET:
WORLD OF WONDER AND DELIGHT

Essential points

When with someone who has Alzheimer's:

- ◆ Learn to see without judgement.
- ◆ Enter his world; leave yours behind.
- ◆ Learn to play.
- ◆ Look for the feelings and emotions behind his words.
- ◆ Be mindful of your own body language and gestures, and what that communicates.

> *I am not in my perfect mind,*
> *Methinks I should know you, and know this man*
> *Yet I am doubtful; for I am mainly ignorant what*
> *place this is;*
> *And all the skill I have remembers not these garments;*
> *Nor I know not where I did lodge last night.*
>
> Shakespeare, *King Lear*

Enclosed within his white merry walker,* Ben wanders from one end of the hall to the other, back and forth, again and again, without ever tiring. Wearing his beige hat tilting to one side, he smiles and grins at the world he sees around him. And that world is an amazing place! His steps are small and quick, as he gazes straight ahead at the long hallway with its cacophony of sounds — beeping call lights, voices, shouts and cries, mixing with another sound, equally as discordant yet subtle: the buzzing sound of fluorescent lights, buzzing without end. With a twinkle in his eyes, Ben's expression is always one of curiosity and wonder as he looks ahead, without turning his gaze to admire the colorful paintings strategically placed on the walls to add a spark of beauty to these otherwise drab hallways, where residents sit in their wheelchairs daily lined up on both sides.

He is no longer able to communicate with words, but his expressions speak louder than words. He does not stop smiling, and often he will laugh. Sometimes it is a jolly *ho, ho, ho*, Santa Clause-like laugh. Other times it is a chuckle that seems to say, *if only you could see what I see, if only you knew what I know*. It is like *his secret*, and if only we knew, we too might wander around smiling and laughing unceasingly. I only wish I knew what he was seeing. I wish I could experience his world for just one moment in time, experience whatever must tickle him on the inside.

Wherever he is in space and time, I doubt it is unpleasant. I believe it is more unpleasant for his family, who cannot understand why or what has happened to their good father, the articulate man, successful in his profession as a banker, who had, as they say, *all his marbles*. But when I watch him, he seems perfectly content wandering around, stopping from time to time, if something or someone captures his fancy. Then he will stare, as if to ponder some hidden message, to decipher a deeper meaning. Sometimes 30 or 40 minutes will pass, and he is still there.

Every once in a while, if you try to talk with him, he will mumble a few inarticulate words while shaking his head, or bobbing it up and down. He could be saying, *I am doing fine, just fine, and you?* Sometimes he will stand outside of another resident's room, just peering inside, studying it in great detail. Often he comes to my office and parks his merry walker outside, gazing within. If only he could get in–it's just a little too big to fit through an average-sized doorway — but he tries anyway, as if by perseverance, his walker will magically tear down the wall for him to enter. I go over to him and ask how he is doing, but he says nothing, only smiles, so I ask him again. He keeps smiling and then starts laughing and laughing.

Ben is especially responsive to an older woman, another resident's wife. She flirts with him, and he follows her from place to place. She has managed a great task – getting him to wheel her husband's wheelchair back to his room. Walking alongside Ben, she guides the journey. He responds to those he knows. He may not know who they are exactly, but their presence, their way of being with him, the familiarity of their face or their touch, makes him remember.

One day, just before the sun set, he wandered to the glass exit door, wearing his hat and beige trousers matching his plaid shirt, except this time, I had to rub my eyes to see if what I was seeing was real. His pants were down below his knees, revealing his white rump! But that didn't seem to faze him. He just kept smiling at the world outside, with its parking lot, tree-lined street, and sun setting behind verdant hills. Maybe he was simply curious, or maybe he saw the world in a way I couldn't. Maybe he had answers we don't have, the world he saw more real than the one most of us see. Or maybe he was just enjoying that moment of being.

* Merry walker is a plastic self-enclosed walker to protect someone from falling.

PART IV

THE POWER OF TOUCH

11

MASSAGE FOR HER MOTHER? REALLY?

Essential points

- ◆ Think out of the box, and try something new.
- ◆ Trust your intuition.
- ◆ Touch is vital to feeling alive!
- ◆ Use massage, Therapeutic Touch, Reiki, and other forms of touch therapy.

Nothing is so healing as the human touch.

Bobbie Fischer

Andrea was skeptical. Massage for her mother? Ruth never had a massage in her life. Could massage really help? She could be difficult. She didn't like most people, and most people didn't like her. She was always complaining, never happy, nothing was ever right. She could be highly critical and morose at times. And everything was becoming so costly—the assisted living community where she recently moved, her companion/caregiver, her psychotherapist — and now a massage therapist?

But massage was highly recommended by Ruth's psychotherapist, who intuitively sensed that massage would be the perfect adjunct therapy in helping her deal with her depression, anxiety and isolation.

Ruth's face had settled into a permanent frown. The therapist thought massage would help lift and soften her facial muscles while lightening the heaviness in her heart. Massage would bring more equanimity and relaxation, as well as flexibility in her fingers that had become rigid.

Although skeptical, Andrea decided to try it—at least once.

I was delighted. One of my greatest loves is in working with clients who struggle with depression, isolation, and loneliness because there the need for touch and connection is the greatest. To experience a positive heartfelt shift in another human being is what inspires me most of all.

Though eager to meet Ruth, I was not quite sure what to expect, but I went without any preconceived ideas. My intention was to bring my full presence, with a caring, compassionate heart.

When I knocked on the door, she yelled out, "Who is it?" in a husky and stern voice. When I replied, she told me to open the door and come in. Her room was sparse: eggshell walls with no decorations or clocks anywhere. She lay on her bed in her two-room apartment, wide awake with unkempt gray hair and thick black glasses, looking gruff. For a moment, I wondered if she even wanted me there, but when she asked me where and how I would do the massage, I knew she wanted me to stay. I suggested different ways of working with her, and she opted for sitting upright in her living room chair. She got up, grabbed her walker and took a few steps to the chair. Although it was a hot California autumn day, she wore a gray angora cardigan that I helped her take off, then I removed her glasses and placed them carefully on the coffee table.

I began by gently holding the back of her neck and forehead for a few moments so she would get used to my hands. Though stiff, she did not resist. I held the intention of helping to facilitate whatever inner healing was needed. I focused on bringing peace and love. After pausing with a breath, I added something else — joy — then let my fingers sweep lightly across her forehead and cheeks, feeling the deep set worry lines beneath my fingertips, the hollowness within her cheeks, the bumpy roughness of her chin, stopping to press lightly pressure points along the way. I felt her focusing on the sensations she was experiencing. She was completely present and open as the tension in her face softened beneath my touch.

As I continued massaging her shoulders, her neck, and arms, she sighed a long breath out, the kind of breath that told me she was letting go and releasing tension. It was like entering another space, peeling away another layer to go deeper. She kept her eyes closed for the duration; nothing could disturb the kind of present and peaceful state of mind she seemed to enter. We worked in silence.

It was quiet outside except for the occasional sound of a distant car, footsteps in the courtyard below and subdued voices in conversation. The afternoon sun shone through the bare window. Every subtle movement of touch, glide, stroke became a meditation as the minutes unfolded.

Not everyone has the ability to be as still, silent, and present as Ruth. That was part of why I especially enjoyed working with her. When our session was coming to a close, I placed one hand on her heart, the other on the back of her neck and silently offered my wish that her heart would be light, and peace, healing, love, and joy would flow through her. Then I knelt down, and placed my hand on her hand to let her know that our session was over. Startled, she opened her eyes like a snoozing cat suddenly awakened in the midst of a pleasant dream. "Time is up, you mean?" she said in her husky voice.

I couldn't help but smile, charmed by her response. I liked her, even though on the surface she might appear gruff. "I can come back, if you'd like me to," I said, thinking about how happy her daughter would be knowing how different she now appeared: her eyes sparkled, and her face and shoulders had softened. She looked much more at peace.

"I'll talk to my daughter. I'd like you to come back soon."

And as I was about to leave, she turned around with something pressing to say: "Thank you." Her words were heartfelt, and I was touched.

When I spoke with Andrea the following day, she was so pleased. "What did you do? She loved you and your massage! I'd like you to continue working with her twice a month." Ruth's therapist later told me Ruth's muscles did in fact seem to soften. "She smiles more now, and seems more easy-going, relaxed, and friendly."

It has been over a year now that I've been working with Ruth, and she continues to enjoy her bi-weekly massages. She now has a big round clock and some prints decorating her wall, a cute little ceramic dog napping on the floor, that almost looks real, some pictures of her family on the table, including the newest addition — a great granddaughter — of whom she is so happy and proud. And when we come to the end of our session, she continues to respond like the snoozing cat who has suddenly been startled, "Time is up, you mean?" Each time I can't help but smile.

"But I'll be back soon."

Further thoughts

Touch is healing and connects us in ways that words cannot. Touch goes beyond language, age, religion, and condition. When touch is done with caring, compassionate intention, it becomes a gift.

I am continually amazed by how healing massage can be. By "healing" I don't mean that people are suddenly cured of all their ills, but that some deep inner shift occurs that can be restorative and life changing. Some examples are: the person feels more at peace, more loved and cared for with a deeper sense of purpose, and has an overall sense of well-being. I have also worked with elders who have never had a massage and didn't think they would even like one, but discovered it is one of the highlights in their lives, something they look forward to on an ongoing basis.

The beauty of massage is it can work with anyone—no matter how fragile or incoherent the person may seem — as long as it is done with care and skill. Massage can be especially effective with people who have Alzheimer's by lessening anxiety and helping to bring a sense of connection and validation. Reiki or Therapeutic Touch can benefit elders who are extremely fragile or on hospice. Touch therapy in whatever form is a wonderful tool.

Touch therapy knows no bounds. I work with a Persian lady who does not speak English. She suffers from pains in her arms and hands and has a tremor in one hand. She speaks to me in her native language. Though I don't understand Farsi, I understand the warmth and appreciation that her words convey. I work gently with her, and when her hand begins to tremor, I simply hold it, using Reiki, and after a few moments it stops shaking. She smiles and kisses me. Love always shines in her eyes.

Suggestions for creating engaging and inspiring activities

♦ Use touch therapy and a caring touch more often with your elders. Touch therapy refers to any number of therapeutic touch modalities administered by a trained professional. Some of those modalities include, but are not limited to, massage, acupressure, Therapeutic Touch, and Reiki.

For family caregivers

♦ Give the gift of an ongoing massage by a professional massage therapist.

♦ Give more back rubs and shoulder rubs to your loved one.

♦ Hug, hold hands, and cuddle more, when and if appropriate.

A POEM FOR ANNA

May the work of your hands be a sign of gratitude and reverence to the human condition.

Mahatma Gandhi

My hand touched your hand
when I saw your distress
as you sat with your elbow bent,
head in your hand.

You were tall, slender,
        but your belly was enormous,
filled with fluids
like a big water balloon
that you could not burst
to drain and free
but had to hold in discomfort,
preventing you from proper sleep,
ease and peace.

It could have been me.
We were the same age,
            just over 50
but it was you.

I asked if you'd like a gentle massage
for you seemed so sweet, kind, caring,
beautiful, radiant and too young
to leave this world.

You weren't wizened
like Ella, Margaret, Maria, or Sue,
who were at the nurse's station too,
waiting … .
                    waiting …
                                waiting …
for something …
                        anything…
relief, medication, a visit,
lunch, dinner, a doctor's visit,
                                    waiting…

perhaps thinking
what one resident repeatedly said,
"This is the last stop, isn't it?
We're all waiting now,
just waiting."

You just didn't seem to fit.

I wanted nothing more than to console you,
To bring you some relief.
And I wanted to ask,

have you made peace?
are you ready?

It could have been me,
but it was you,
lifting your head,
your gray-blue eyes
like water reflecting light
of some vague longing,
the mystery of sadness, pain, death,
God.

"Yes … a gentle massage
would be lovely."

I touched your shoulders and neck,
silent prayers flowing
through my fingertips,
stroking softly,
sweeping fluidly,
humbly
feeling bones
more than muscle and skin.

And I wanted to ask,
did you accomplish your dreams?
are you afraid?

but I did not speak,

I thought of your dear mother
whom I massaged
when I saw how broken she was.
She kept mentioning your son,
his first year in college.

And I wanted to ask
who is he,
how is he?
but I do not speak.

I only touched with praying hands,
desiring to bring comfort,
healing of the heart,
pulsing and breathing
gathering in sparks
of One Breath,
            one Being
                  your Light touched my Light.

Tenderness.
           Touch.
                  Healing.

Then I held one palm to your forehead,
the other to your heart and whispered
"I hope you feel better."

You opened your eyes
with a twinkle
like a child who just received
some wondrous gift,

"This is the first time in a long time
I feel this much comfort and relief.
I can lie down now
and fall asleep … fall asleep … thank you."

We were two lives passing,
a few holy moments in time.

13

MAKING THE ROUNDS:
HEALING HANDS IN SKILLED NURSING

Essential points

♦ Create a healing environment for your elders.
♦ Touch is vital to feeling alive.
♦ Use massage, Therapeutic Touch, Reiki, and other forms of touch therapy.

The residents anticipate my coming and ask the activity director, *when is the massage lady coming? Is it today?* I'm there twice a month. Some residents wait inside the activity room in wheelchairs or with walkers, scattered about at the tables and in between. Some residents are lined up in the hallway. I stop to greet each one before entering the room.

I turn off the television, blaring the news of the day, and replace it with soft music. Lulling flute and piano, the ting, tang ring and chime of Tibetan bowls. The atmosphere begins to change, creating a space for healing, stirring waves that nourish the heart, uplift the spirit, and shift the inner landscape into light.

I take my magical elixirs: calming lavender, rejuvenating rose, stimulating ylang ylang, and rosemary for sore muscles. Making eye contact, I greet each resident with a light touch on the hand or arm. Betty tells me how happy she is to see me and how much the massage has helped her stiff neck and arthritic hands. For 10-15 minutes I massage her shoulders, neck, arms, and hands. She closes her eyes and takes in the experience fully. She is hard of hearing so when I am finished, I tap her lightly and write on a small white board with a marker, "Thank you, I hope this was helpful."

She nods her head, "You've helped me so much, if you only knew."

Then, I go to Mrs. Stein, who gets highly agitated and will often repeat the same words again and again. Over the past months, she has also repeated the same story.

"They came over on a boat from Ellis island, my mother says, they lived down the street, and Mr. Brown killed her ... he killed her ... they came over on a boat from Ellis island, my mother says and Mr. Brown killed her."

Her eyes have a distant glaze of someone who is in another world from the past, but when I touch her hand, make eye contact and ask, "How are you today, Mrs. Stein?" she becomes present and leaves behind the world of Ellis Island and Mr. Morris.

Smiling, she says, "I am good, thank you, you are a nice lady, thank you, thank you for coming today." I ask if I may massage her shoulders and neck. She looks at me, puzzled, not knowing what I mean, so I take her hand and begin gently massaging and say, like this, "Massage, may I massage your hands?"

"Yes, yes, yes," she exclaims. After working with her a few moments, she becomes silent, a rare occasion. The caregivers peek inside the room and stand oohing and aahing. They are not used to seeing Mrs. Stein so calm.

When I finish, she says, "Thank you, you are a nice lady. The nice lady came to see us today, she is a real nice lady. Thank you, thank you, nice lady."

I walk over to Mrs. Smith, whose feet are propped up on the foot rest of her wheelchair. Holding her hands over the crocheted blanket that covers her, she tilts her head and lifts the corner of her mouth in a smile. She does not speak, but often expresses her affection by caressing my head and face. I hold her feet, then her hand, then the back of her neck and heart, and send loving energy through her. There have been times when I couldn't get to her in a timely fashion, and with sad eyes she looked towards me, lifting up her arms. I couldn't resist.

Bob, a small frail but frenetic man wearing a white T-shirt, walks back and forth, unable to sit still. I take his hand and lead him to a chair while he asks, "Where are you taking me? I'm looking for my mother. Did you see her? Can you help me?"

I tell him she will be here soon. "I'll give you a massage while we wait for her. Just listen to the music."

"Why are you going to give me a massage?"

"I think you'll like it, and it'll help you relax while we wait for your mother."

Bob is not easy. He sits down and forgets about our conversation and asks the man sitting at the table if he's seen his mother. The man says no. Slowly, gently, I begin massaging Bob's shoulders, as he says, "Hey, this is great! I've never had anybody do this for me before, not even my mother. I must be a nice person for you to do this for me."

"You are very nice, Bob."

"This is great! You're even better looking than my mother!"

Bob's shoulders begin to soften. The tense muscles of his frowning face transform and soften. He closes his eyes and becomes quiet.

Francis wanders in the room with the glazed eyes of someone who is far away. She has Alzheimer's and, like Bob, she is an agitated wanderer, but she cannot speak English, only French.

The activity director asks if I can massage her when I am through with Bob, but I never get to her, because Tiko, a Korean lady who also doesn't speak English, has been observing me and begins massaging Francis's shoulders, neck, arms and hands as she keeps studying me in imitation and speaking in Korean. Tiko wears a loose frock and white anklets; her hair is a mass of gray and black curls. Although she is hunched over, she walks quickly and nimbly. When she massages Francis, it is with the same vigor. The staff come to watch Tiko in the midst of her massage.

I have seen Tiko pray in her room. Her side of the room holds a silent holiness, with a small statue of a mediating Buddha sitting on a cloth covered table with prayer beads and scrolls. I have also seen her in the garden wandering among the flowers and trees. Sometimes I wonder what passes through her mind when she stops in front of the same oak tree again and again. She looks closely at it as if for the first time, touching its trunk, as if it is a fascinating mystery, pausing and running her fingers in between the rough edges of bark, and with a sense of awe and wonder gazing up at its branches.

Out in the garden, Joseph sometimes sits in his wheelchair next to the bird bath. Other times he is inside the activity room waiting to be touched. He's had a stroke and lost use of one side of his body. His arm and hand flop over his lap, as if he wishes it were not there, or as if it were some alien appendage that doesn't belong to him. He is angry at himself and others but especially at the arm which he can no longer use so he must rely on everyone for help. He is frustrated, too, because he cannot communicate his needs, though he tries.

He does not like me to massage the affected side of his body. I speak softly, letting him know, moment by moment, what I am doing, going from shoulder to arm to elbow and hand, always reassuring him that I know he doesn't like to be massaged on the right side. The massage softens his spirit, lightens and brightens his being. He even pauses and smiles warmly. When he knows I will be there, he looks for me.

Holding a worn-out teddy bear, Dalia sits next to the glass door overlooking the garden, with her hair tied back in a bun, with a tumor growing on her forehead the size of a golf ball and repeats over and over again, "How I want to be a good mother, how I want to be a good mother, I tried so hard."

"It's so nice to see you, Dalia, and you are a good mother. You've done so much good. And the children love you." I massage her hand gently. With her sparkling blue eyes, she gazes at me, as if taking me in, yet simultaneously lost in another world.

"Oh, yes, the children were happy," she says so casually, as if in a routine conversation with a close friend over a cup of tea.

"Yes, they were happy and you're so good."

I see Carla, in her tiger print pullover and slippers down the hallway wheeling herself with one arm and holding a cup of coffee with the other. She tells me how much the massage helped her shoulder last week, with all its knots and kinks. We have our usual chit chat, which always leads to something deeper, more personal. "Can you tell me how to be more present? I struggle with it, but it's hard, my mind won't shut off. I worry. I'm unhappy. I'm angry. I'm frustrated. All these things that I can't stop, but if I were more present, things might change. Do you know how to be more present?"

I'm astounded that she has asked me this question in a place where there is so much suffering. A wise and noble question. Presence is powerful. "Try to focus on the breath, going in and out, feeling each subtle movement of air going into your nostrils, feeling it at the tip of your nose and down into the belly as your belly rises. Focus on the breath going in and out. Let your thoughts come and go. Don't be attached to them, don't cling, simply let them come and go." I guide her in a meditative breath practice, then massage her neck and shoulders, her upper back, feeling her breath rising and falling beneath my touch. Presence fills the space with timeless mystery. I knead gently, going down her arms, as she continues to breathe and when I finish, I ask her if the breathing was helpful and she tells me it was.

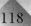

Then I ask, "Are you feeling sad about something in particular?"

"It's my new roommate. She's not a nice person. She yells at me. She puts the television on too loud. She lays awake at night and keeps me up. She curses at me if I ask her to lower the volume. I'm exhausted the next day and next day and the next because the same thing happens again and again."

"Did you say anything to anyone here, like the social worker?"

"No."

"I think you should."

Two months later, she moves into another room with a roommate who is much more genial. The change uplifts her tremendously.

Some residents have been here for years or months. Others pass through quickly, either because they recovered from a fall or surgery or are on hospice. The Director of Nursing asks me to visit John, who has much physical discomfort and pain and might benefit from a light massage. He is on hospice, and has accepted his death, does not fight it and is at peace. He knows it will come any day.

For about six weeks, throughout the day, he wakes up and falls asleep. With time he sleeps more and wakes up less, eats less, drinks less, has a need to talk less and his dosage of morphine increases. Each day I hope he will be there. I have become fond of him because he seems so thoughtful and gentle, intelligent and kind. I enjoy the sweetness of his presence and think of him every morning during my prayers. *May he be at peace and free from suffering.*

He becomes frailer each time I see him, so frail that when I touch him it is with a feather light touch that is closer to simple holding. My hand touches his forehead, stays there quietly, unobtrusively, or sometimes near his heart. I send him peace, peace, peace. One day as I crept up beside him ever so gently, he opened his eyes and thought I was his kitty, Minerva. He smiled, then closed his eyes and fell asleep. His daughter came in one day shortly after I worked with him, and came out of his room in search of the person who had just been with him to say thank you. "You've brought so much relief to my father." She was in tears, distraught that her father was dying, yet also so grateful that her father was being given some relief.

Sometimes I wonder if I am doing enough, if I am really helping as much as I'd like, and when I hear someone say something like this, I am happy. That is what I am there for. That is my work.

When I finish with my work here and walk out the double glass doors at the entrance, there is always a little bit of sadness knowing that death is here, and I never know if John or any of the other residents will be there the next time I come, yet there is an even bigger sense of inspiration and joy—knowing that I was able to relieve some suffering, even if in a small way. I was touched, and I touched. That gives me great satisfaction.

Further thoughts

Some potential benefits of massage:

- ◆ Improves circulation

- ◆ Lessens dependence on medication

- ◆ Releases endorphins—the amino acids that work as the body's natural pain killer

- ◆ Boosts immune system by stimulating lymph flow—the body's natural defense system

- ◆ Improves sleep

- ◆ Improves concentration

- ◆ Increases joint flexibility

- ◆ Lessens depression and anxiety

- ◆ Encourages overall well-being

Research on massage shows:

- **Parkinson's patients** may have fewer tremors and less muscle and joint stiffness

- **Arthritis sufferers** may have fewer aches and less stiffness and pain

- **High blood pressure patients** may demonstrate lower diastolic blood pressure, anxiety, and stress hormones

- **Alzheimer's patients** may exhibit reduced pacing, irritability, and restlessness

- **Stroke patients** may show less anxiety and lower blood pressure

Recommended reading on massage:

I highly recommend an insightful article in the March 5, 2015 issue of the *New Yorker* called "The Power of Touch," by Maria Konnikova. She cites the 30 + years of research done by Dr. Tiffany Field, the head of the Touch Research Institute at the University of Miami's Miller School of Medicine.

In a series of studies by Dr. Field, "one group of elderly participants received regular, conversation-filled social visits while another received social visits that also included massage; the second group saw emotional and cognitive benefits over and above those of the first ... Touch can lower blood pressure, heart rate, and cortisol levels, stimulate the hippocampus, and drive the release of a host of hormones and neuropeptides that have been linked to positive and uplifting emotions. The physical effects of touch are far-reaching."

Suggestions for creating engaging and inspiring activities

♦ Consider starting a massage therapy program for your elders.

♦ If the budget does not allow for a program, bring in a massage therapist who can make him or herself available to interested residents. Inform families by giving them the massage therapist's brochure or card.

Choosing a massage therapist:

♦ Not every massage therapist is alike, nor every massage. Find someone who brings the best to your elders.

♦ Consider this: Does your elder seem more at peace during and after the massage? More uplifted? Is there a positive change in the general atmosphere of the room?

♦ Look for a therapist who has been trained properly with a background in geriatric massage, who understands the aging body and the conditions, both physical and mental, that may arise, and who knows what it is like to reside in long-term care.

♦ Some questions to ask a massage therapist:

• What is your background?

• Where have you been trained? For how long? (It is good to have at least 500 hours of training.)

• Are you state certified?

• Has your training included geriatric massage?

• How long have you been in practice?

BE PRESENT AND LOVE...
WITHOUT WANT OR EXPECTATION

Essential points

♦ Create a healing environment for your elders.
♦ Touch is vital to feeling alive.
♦ Use massage, Therapeutic Touch, Reiki, and other forms of touch therapy.

> *To love ... implies caring for, knowing, responding, affirming, enjoying: the person, the tree, the painting, the idea. It implies bringing to life, increasing his/her/its aliveness. It is a process, self-renewing and self-increasing.*
>
> Erich Fromm

I never saw them often, or at least not during the first year I worked there, so I did not know much about them at all. Theirs seemed to be a private world separate from the rest of the community, with their own furniture, fluffy and colorful bed covers, and framed photographs adorning the walls, making their room cozy, quaint, and homey. Rarely did they come out of their room, so it wasn't until later that I really got to know them through my work as a massage therapist.

During that time, I discovered that they were well cared for. Their son, Michael, was always trying to figure out ways of bringing more comfort, joy, and pleasure into their lives, and it showed in everything he did. He had two of the kindest, most loving private duty caregivers. Nellie and Sam took care of his parents as if they were their own mother and father. Michael also brought in a large screen TV, with the intention that his parents would be able to watch some of their favorite movies on a nice large screen. Neither one could walk, so they spent part of their day in bed; George, in his bed, and Ginger in her bed, close to each other yet separated by a couple of night tables; and part of their day out of bed, when their caregivers lifted them up out of bed with a lift, then dressed them nicely before sitting them down in their very soft and cozy reclining chairs that Michael had brought in for them.

Nellie took care of Ginger, and made sure that she had lipstick, mascara, and blush on, that her nails and hair were done, that she was showered and fresh, wearing a clean set of clothes, something comfortable like stretch cotton pants and a top, with some delicate frill or flower on it, something pretty and feminine. That was what Ginger had been used to, except in those younger days her attire would have been much more glamorous and sexy.

George was dressed in his usual manner, which was always subtler, quieter and less bold in color than hers: brown, beige or navy blue pants and a simple polo shirt or plaid. In their younger days, she had been the gregarious social butterfly, who liked dressing up and drinking martinis, sometimes one too many, while he had been the teetotaler, the quiet one, who preferred staying at home with a cup of a tea. Yet he loved her, and she adored him.

Before working with them privately, I had very little contact with them. Usually it was when the weather was warm and sunny when Nellie and Sam took them outside for a stroll or to sit in the garden. Like the grand old couple, with their sunglasses and sun hats on, his in beige, hers in hot pink, they were wheeled down the hallway, tucked comfortably into their wheelchairs with extra padding, laps covered with fluffy blankets, hers in white, his in navy blue, and legs propped up for circulation. No one really knew much about them, except for their caregivers, and of course their son.

Sometimes I caught glimpses of them through the window, where they sat in the garden near my office — Ginger in her hot pink sun hat, matching hot pink pants, and white top with a big, hot pink, sparkly daisy-like flower in the middle. With amusement, I also noticed that whenever Ginger saw one caregiver in particular, her pudgy yet shapely legs squirmed in the chair, like the legs of a squirming baby, as a big smile lit up her face, accompanied by eye batting, coquettish laughter, and an endless stream of murmurs and coos.

What did she say? No one could quite understand. There was speculation, nothing definite or concrete, yet it was clear that everyone who knew her knew she had a special affection for this one particular caregiver – a young, dashing and handsome Filipino who sat in the garden often with the elder man he cared for. He flirted right back with her. I could not help putting down whatever paperwork I was doing to enjoy the flirtation between Ginger and the dark, handsome caregiver.

Meanwhile, Sam was busy engaging George with jokes and banter, which typically would have been enough to occupy his attention (as I came to discover later), but this time, he was struggling to turn his head to view the dalliance. Because his range of motion was severely limited, it was never an easy task to turn his head. He had to shift slowly and carefully the whole upper part of his body. He had an uncommon brain disorder that affects movement, similar to Parkinson's, as well as severe arthritis that made both his hands clench up into tight fists. If he were able to speak, I wondered what he might have said, but George did not speak, except on rare occasions.

Unlike his wife, George was fairly lucid. He was aware of everything happening around him. Ginger was already in the advanced stages of Alzheimer's, yet if she was having a good day, and the handsome, young caregiver was around, magic happened. That was only on a good day and at a particular time of day, usually early or late morning and early afternoon.

When the sun started to go down, there was a sudden shift in Ginger. In elder care communities, sunset is the time of day when those with dementia, especially Alzheimer's, become extremely confused, disoriented, and irritable. This condition is known as *sundowning*. Ginger cried incessantly during that time. It was as if while the sun set, she slipped into another world, a world that seemed impossible to break through.

Later, I would often hear Nellie say, *oh mama, mama, I only wish I knew what was making you cry*, while taking Ginger's face endearingly into her hands. The first actual encounter I ever had with Ginger, before working with her, was during a brief time when Nellie left work early because her family was visiting from the Philippines. Not wanting to leave Ginger in the room without anyone to assist her (George's caregiver was also away in the Philippines visiting his family,) Nellie brought her into the hallway near the nurse's station, where Ginger continued to wail incessantly, although Nellie reassured her as best as she could.

George would be just fine staying in his room eating quietly with one of the community's caregivers feeding him. George was not difficult to assist. He wasn't very demanding, and although he needed assistance for everything from going to the toilet to eating to being turned in bed and dressed, he did not require much else, as his wife did. She needed special attention.

When I first saw her sitting in the hallway, it was the end of a long, exhausting day. I had not eaten lunch and worked longer than my usual seven hour day. I was irritable and cranky. Sitting in the practically empty hallway, too tired to pick myself up in that moment to go home, I saw Ginger, sitting kitty corner across from me, next to the nurse's station. Normally, it was quiet around that time of day. I was hoping it would be, especially on that day, but it wasn't.

Ginger's high pitched cry drilled in my head, reverberating within the intense pounding that was already there. Puzzled by her, I stared and noticed that her face was without emotion, her eyes filled with a glossy emptiness, focused on some distant place. It was almost like a mechanical gesture, yet it was loud and incessant, mixed with unintelligible utterances, without one moment to stop for a breath, or so it seemed.

I stared at her, noticing her pudgy red cheeks, her curly white hair, disheveled and standing straight up on her head, and I thought to myself, *Why are you crying like that? It is annoying! Excruciatingly annoying … Stop it! Stop it!* I wanted to shout, *Stop your whining already. I have had enough!*

Of course I did not say those words, but I thought them, and I was surprised when suddenly she turned her head and looked in my direction. Not only did she seem to become more agitated, but she cried even louder. Was it me, or was it just coincidence? I didn't know, but on further thought, I decided it was best to call it a day and go home.

On my way home that evening, I felt guilty for having had those thoughts, yet I also reminded myself that I am only human, and any human who is overworked or tired, especially from working in skilled nursing, is not able to give her best. Caregivers are constantly giving, constantly moving and exerting physical strength and energy. Overwork and exhaustion are not uncommon. A 40-hour work week is the bane of skilled nursing. Taking care of oneself is important. Balance among work, family, pleasure and rest is essential.

Tomorrow, I thought, *will be a new day. I will be well rested and fresh. I will try something different. I will sit with her, not apart from her, but with her and try to console her in some way. In what way? What will I do?* I wondered… *Be present and love…* were the words I heard from a voice within. *Be present and love…*

The following day when Nellie left early for the day and brought Ginger into the hallway, she was whining loudly, making agitated motions with her legs and hands. *What could be making her cry like that?* I wondered. *Was she remembering some part of her past, some unresolved piece of the past? Was it the medication? What was it?*

Quietly, I sat with her and began talking softly and slowly in a very calm and soothing manner, letting her know that Nellie would be back in the morning, and that we were all there to help her. Then I tried massaging her neck and shoulders lightly. Even that did not seem to work. She wailed again like the previous evening. Her gaze was focused somewhere far off in the distance, as if she did not see me, hear me, or know I existed. She was in her own world, and there was no room for me to slip in, so that evening I let her be, but I did not give up.

The rest of the week I kept trying while hearing those words within, *be present and love… be present and love.* One day I even tried gently stroking her forehead, which I thought might have a particularly calming effect. I imagined peace flowing through my fingertips, yet it seemed to make her cry even more. I thought if I were some dark and handsome young man, then maybe. Yet I am not so sure that would even work, at least not at that hour.

Shortly thereafter, Nellie's family returned to the Philippines and with Nellie now staying later, there was no need for Ginger to sit by the nursing station. Weeks had passed without my seeing her or George. It was winter. Both started to decline, but by spring their son, Michael, forever thinking of ways to bring more pleasure into their lives, had an idea. Hire a massage therapist! A weekly massage for them both, something they can really look forward to, perhaps the one last remaining pleasure, Michael thought.

With my background in both elder care and massage, I was just the person to do it. I had been working at a spa for several years. Although my clients there were mainly strong, agile men and women, a good part of my training had been in working with frail adults at the end of their life, an area that I really intended to focus on, so this was the perfect opportunity for me. Yet I must confess that the first thought that flashed through my mind was the memory of that one day while sitting across from Ginger, and of the frustrating days that followed. I grew concerned. *What if I still cannot get through? What if it is more of the same thing? Will she even enjoy it? Will she cry the whole time and shake in agitation and make unintelligible utterances endlessly? ... Don't worry, don't think so much... Be present and love,* I thought. I wasn't so concerned about George. I wasn't sure *how* he would respond, but somehow I knew he would enjoy it.

Yet at that time I could not have possibly imagined that those weekly sessions would become one of the greatest joys not only in George's life, but in mine, and possibly in Ginger's, although with Ginger, it was harder to tell. The experiences with Ginger were not always consistent. Some days were magical and amazing while other days were not so good. Then there was much frustration. But with George, it was more consistent. Each session was different, yet almost every time George smiled brightly, up until the moment he closed his eyes and fell asleep. Even then, sometimes the smile remained.

George's elation rubbed off on me. I left work smiling, feeling uplifted and energized.

Although George almost never spoke, his eyes expressed another state of being, free of this world's anxieties, discomforts, and endless problems. His eyes were clear and bright, radiant with inner peace. A sense of Presence filled the room as his eyes followed each stroke and glide of my hands, every movement and step that I made around him.

Stillness permeated the hour –not like the stillness I experience in the quiet hours of early morning at home, when the only sounds are an occasional car and the silent buzz within. Here there were all the noises of skilled nursing that are always there: everything from call lights buzzing to fluorescent lights, to chattering voices, to cries of discomfort, to a television blaring from the room next door. Yet it was as if we found our own stillness held within all the noises that were there, that could not be turned off, even with a closed door. During that hour, George was a transformed man. There is something profound and miraculous in seeing that kind of change in someone. By the end of our session, he often let out a long sigh.

Over dinner, I would share with my husband how happy George was, and how exhilarating it was to witness that joy, knowing I was helping to create it. It is one of the highest, most wondrous experiences, especially when it is someone like George, who spends his days in bed, unable to walk or talk, and must rely on a caregiver for all his needs. In short, George had very little left in the way of pleasure or joy.

One day, George surprised me. I heard him say in a faint but audible whisper, "Thank you." I was ecstatic! Although I already knew how appreciative he was, there was something wonderful about hearing him articulate those words. Sam told me that some mornings George did talk, but only every once in a while. Sam also shared with me that whenever Monday came, he would remind George it was the day the massage lady came. George's eyes would light up, his face flushing, and he smiled all day.

I believe that day of anticipation was just as much a bright spot in his life as was the massage itself. Sometimes in spring when Samuel took George out into the garden, he insisted on stopping to see me. He looked up at me with stars in his eyes, like a schoolboy who had a crush on his teacher. It was very sweet, a bright spot in my day, as well as in his.

Ginger was different. It took time for her to get to know me, or at least to become familiar with me and to realize that when she saw me it meant getting a massage. Sometimes I joked with her about being the massage lady who was there to try to make her happy. Sometimes I got her to smile and chuckle. Other times nothing, and many times she simply kept on crying.

Yet there were times when I was surprised and delighted by her responses. These were moments of deep connection, incredibly bright and lucid, as if I had somehow managed to get through. Those moments stand out in my mind most of all because they were so magical … *Be present and love* … with no expected outcomes in mind, surrendering to the present moment, wherever it took us. It was a journey for us both — and a journey for us all, because the caregivers were always present. I was fortunate that they were so helpful in turning George and Ginger over for me, something I would not have been able to do on my own.

I came to truly love Ginger, in her good moments, as well as in her bad, yet often I felt frustrated. She wasn't always responsive, especially when she kept crying with that empty gaze focused on some distant place. There were times when I wanted to shake her and say, *wake up, stop crying, can't you just enjoy this?* Yet there were those light-filled moments of sheer magic that touched my heart deeply. It was as if our two worlds met and stood facing each other, merging into one other.

One day she was especially agitated and annoyingly loud. Just as I was about to honor what I thought might have been her wish not to be touched, I was seized with the sudden impulse to pick up a picture near the bed. It was one of my favorite pictures of her — Ginger in her early 30s perhaps, the eternal glamour queen with her hair curled and thrown onto her head in the typical bouffant of the day, wearing a little black jacket with a leopard print collar.

I am fond of animal prints, so I especially liked that picture, and with enthusiasm I exclaimed, "Wow, what a sexy mama!" I held up the picture in front of her and said it again, "Look, Ginger, look! What a sexy mama you are!" Suddenly, Ginger stopped crying. She paused, looked at the photo, looked at me and began smiling, muttering something which I could not understand, but that seemed playful. She even chuckled. *Wow, I* thought, *this is wonderful!* Wanting to continue in the spirit of play and fun, I joked with her about how she must have been a real tiger in those days!

"Had I been around then, we would have gone out for a couple of glasses of wine. Girls' night out! And girls just want to have fun!" I will never forget that moment because it was as if a light had suddenly melted whatever agitation she felt. Completely calm, she looked right at me, with her eyes meeting mine. She had something to say.

Her blue eyes twinkling, she murmured and cooed unintelligible utterances as if she were telling us her story. Unfortunately, I was not able to understand; neither was Nellie nor Sam. Yet, clearly Ginger was present and alive to that moment. I continued massaging her arm lightly, while bantering with her. Normally I would be quiet while giving a massage, but it seemed more appropriate to use words with Ginger, or at least then. She listened, until she began murmuring and cooing playfully again.

Ten or fifteen minutes must have passed without her crying. Then her gaze went off somewhere in the distance. She remained calm but was no longer present, and by the time I left, she went back to whining, except without the agitation.

I remember another time in the spring, when the hours were longer, and there was still light at six o' clock, which was when I would normally massage them. Ginger's bed was by the window. The blinds were open, so it was possible to still see the courtyard outside with its rose bushes in bloom. A glorious feast of color for the eyes: pink, red, lavender, white, and yellow buds beginning to open, others in full bloom, petals falling to the ground in a silky sweep of dazzling color. The birds were singing and the grass had just been cut, with its fresh scent mixing with the perfumed sweetness of the roses. Ginger was crying again, her eyes, distant and empty, gazing at some invisible point.

I was sitting by the side of her bed, massaging her hands when I said, "I wish I understood why you cry. I wish I understood where you are when you stare off in the distance. I wish I could do something that would suddenly make you stop crying and make you happy."

Ginger turned to me, stopped crying, sighed deeply, and without saying a word, smiled. She bantered about something for a minute or so, then became silent again as she looked outside the window, as if to take in the beauty of the garden in spring. *Wow, this is wonderful*, I thought. Those times were few, and I was ecstatic when they happened. When she was having a bad day, in which almost nothing I did could penetrate, I tried to remind myself of the words I often hear within,

Be present and love … without want, without expectation.

15

TOUCHING TIGER FUR

Essential points

When with someone who has dementia:

- Use the sense of touch more; touch is vital to feeling alive.
- Love unconditionally. The human spirit always recognizes love.
- Don't give up; keep exploring, and be present.
- Search for the hidden gems.
- See the inner light.
- Leave your world behind to enter hers.

> *Though you slip away*
>   *to another world*
> *I will always be here*
>   *for you*
>
> *Though you seem so*
>   *far away*
> *I will never cease*
>   *to love you*

Sometimes you surprise
me with the sunrise
of your splendid soul

Charles Burack

What is it that fascinates me about you, that makes me curious and interested in your world; the world you live in now, woven from dreams and imagination, self-enclosed, unreal to others, yet full, real, and alive to you and only to you; and the other world, the one you once knew before this?

Could it be all the objects in your room that remind me of your past and who you were then: an unframed picture of a monastery nestled within the barren mountains of Tibet hanging on the wall over your bed: a Tibetan prayer wheel, and a little bronze statue of Sarasvati, the Indian goddess of music, scholars, and poets, both surrounded by photos of friends and family in joyous celebration on an old bureau that you yourself brought from home that must have been passed down in your family?

Is it because each time I go into your room, I feel a certain affinity as I look around at the few objects you brought? Or is it how you spend your days dressed in men's attire, sitting with your legs crossed as you engage deeply in some lengthy diagnosis of a client before you, one that I cannot see? That is what it seems, since you were once a professor, psychologist, and researcher. Then again, maybe it is simply the way you always engage in casual conversations with friends or colleagues. I cannot be sure. I only watch and feel a sense of wonder and curiosity about you. When I see you, I think of Freud — or truer to your character, Jung.

I wonder who Lilli, your neighbor in the room next door, is to you. How do you see her? Do you see her as the wiry, rambunctious little lady that she is, irreverent in the best of ways, who wears her hair in thin braids with pink barrettes at the ends? Or does she become someone else? One of your clients perhaps?

I ask, because one day I noticed that you seemed to be in the midst of some lengthy dialogue with her. Yet, when I walked closer, I realized that the conversation did not make any sense. She was having her own conversation that had nothing to do with yours. I heard her say, "Take me to the boys now." Often Lilli spoke about the boys and drinking whisky. She was once a singer. And you were having your own conversation, each with the other, worlds apart, but somehow connecting.

I see vestiges of who you once were: a woman who must have struggled during a time when it was still a man's world. Could it be that I applaud you for what you have done in the world of men, laud your accomplishments, whatever they may have been?

No one ever comes to visit you, except for a nun. I could not help but wonder what happened to all the friends you once knew, the ones in the photos from a happier time? Someone once asked me for advice on how to be with a friend of hers who had Alzheimer's. She confessed that she just did not know what to say or how to behave, and so her visits kept getting postponed into sometime in the future, the future that never came. Could your friends have gone through something similar? And the nun, who is she? I have not yet met her, but I would like to, so that I can ask her questions about you, your life, and fascinating world.

Who would have ever thought that you would be here, in this state-funded care setting with its fetid odors permeating the air, and its cheap plastic-covered chairs, ripped at the edges, with scratched wooden arms? You sit in one of those chairs every day, the same one, just outside your room. Unfortunately, it is not one of those comfortable, softly padded, cloth-covered chairs that you find in some of those grander elder care communities, with their generous endowments that provide the best of everything from food to service, to ambience to programs, to care and comfort. At those places, volunteers are found in abundance, but here they are much fewer, yet it is at places like this where the need is greater.

Why is it that our poor must be denied what is given to others with means? Why is there such a disparity? It concerns and saddens me deeply.

Often I sit next to you. One day, I even reach out for your hand, frail with thick blue veins protruding through pale skin, but it is as if I were not there, and you could not feel my touch; the touch of someone who is fond of you and thinks of you as a kindred spirit. Still, I sit by you anyway and tell you that I adore you and that you fascinate me. I even come to feed you at dinner time. Lifting up the spoon of the pureed food, I place it next to your mouth. Mechanically, you open and swallow while continuing to talk to the imaginary one before you. I, the visible one with the spoon in hand, am invisible to you, but it does not matter. I can love you and be here for you anyway. You are human and so am I, and as humans, we are subject to the same frailties of growing old, becoming sick and dying.

One day I bring in a Tibetan singing bowl. It is a round bowl made of several different metals that makes a sound unlike any other when you glide a wooden mallet around its rim. The Tibetan monks use it as a tool in prayer and meditation. I thought you would like it and even recognize its sound from your past, but when I tap the side of the bowl with the mallet, once, twice, three times, it is as if you could not hear, although it rings like a gong, riding the waves of the air in a call to silence. But I do not give up. I press the mallet to the rim and follow the smooth edge around and around, as its otherworldly sound – arresting and hypnotizing – reverberate through the halls, perking the ears of many. Nurses and caregivers stop what they are doing, curious about the object held in my hand. Everything comes to a standstill. Residents in wheelchairs wheel themselves down the hall, with eyes agog in wonder, and surround us. Even Marge, who never comes out of her room, stands in her doorway. You only stare out into space in front of you.

But I still do not give up. Once the crowd disperses, I pause from playing to tell you about my travels to Nepal, something I thought you would have appreciated. I share with you the story of how while hiking in the mountains, I heard a sound that was so alluring and haunting that I followed it to the village below, where I discovered what it was: a singing bowl. I was so mesmerized by its beauty that I spent the entire day there listening to the bowl maker tell me stories and lore of their ancient history. But each time I look at you, there is nothing, no response, not even a hint. I play the bowl again, hoping the second time you might hear, but it is as if there were an invisible wall between us, and you could not hear me or the sound of the bowl. It is as if there were no object, a sacred one at that, even near you. Still, every day I try something new, hoping that I will reach or touch you in some way.

One day in December, when the northern California air is crisp and cool, I wear my warm faux fur tiger coat. As I make my rounds to say goodbye, I come to you. This time you are not in your usual chair, but walking back and forth in the hallway. You notice me for the first time, but it is the coat that makes you see me. You run your fingers through the fur, and its softness excites you.

I could see it on your face as you exclaim, "ohhhh, oooooo, ahhh, yes, I like that, I like that very much, I like the way that feels." You even look right at me and say, almost under your breath, "You're here observing, aren't you?" Studying me, sizing me up, you then say, "I know you are one of those girlie girls, aren't you, but you're a good kind of girlie girl."

I am stunned! *I finally got through!* I would have never guessed that it would have been the coat. *Oh boy! I will wear this coat each and every day, even in the summer!* And every evening when I am about to leave, I do wear it and take your hand so that you can feel the soft texture, but it does not always work. When it does, you are present with me, present to the touch of tiger fur. But most days, it is as if you could not feel, and as if I still do not exist. But it doesn't matter, I will love you anyway.

Further thoughts

The elder in this story was correctly diagnosed with Lewy Body dementia after having been misdiagnosed with Alzheimer's. According to the Lewy Body Dementia Association, it is important to be diagnosed correctly for two reasons:

♦ People with LBD may respond more favorably to certain dementia medications than people with Alzheimer's, allowing for early treatment that may improve or extend the quality of life for both the person with LBD and their caregiver.

♦ Many people with LBD respond more poorly to certain medications for behavior and movement than people with Alzheimer's or Parkinson's, sometimes with dangerous or permanent side effects.

Some symptoms that differentiate from Alzheimer's include:

♦ Unpredictable levels of cognitive ability

♦ More attention or alertness

♦ Changes in walking or movement

♦ Visual hallucinations

♦ A sleep disorder called REM sleep behavior disorder, in which people physically act out their dreams

♦ Severe sensitivity to medications for hallucinations

HEY, HEY, HEY
TRANSFORMS INTO
YES, YES, YES

Essential Points

♦ Use touch more; touch is vital to feeling alive!
♦ Provide choices that encourage, invite, and support your elders.
♦ Think out of the box, and try something new.
♦ Don't let judgments taint your vision.
♦ Search for hidden gems.
♦ Create community. It has the potential to be a powerful source of healing, growth, and nurturance for your elders.

I imagine that yes is the only living thing.

E. E. Cummings

"Hey, hey, hey," Fran would call out in her raspy voice with her hand shaking, pointing to nearly everyone who passed by, yet she had this air about her of someone who did not want to be bothered. Fran sat in the hallway in her wheelchair, her feet tucked into softly padded slippers, her wiry hair always disheveled. Fran was a woman of very few words. *Hey, hey, hey* was one of them.

I was affectionate with nearly all the residents I worked with, but there were always a few who I sensed did not want to be touched. She was one of them, so I did not shower her with affection. Neither was she one for showing emotion, except for displeasure. Rarely did she smile or laugh. Often she made faces that expressed her displeasure, yet she was harmless and not unkind.

Her *hey, hey, hey* always struck me as funny. No one ever quite knew what she wanted. Joking with her, in a playful tone, I would say, "Hey, hey, hey. What do you want? Who are you calling for?"

"I want you."

"And what can I do for you?" I'd ask. Turning her hands over to reveal her palms, she would say, "I don't know what I want."

Sometimes I would say, "I love you anyway." Her response was always the same. She would wave me away, as if she did not believe me. Still, whenever she called out *hey, hey hey,* I rushed to her side and bantered about her *hey, hey, hey.*

One day when I asked her how she was doing, she shrugged her shoulders as if to say, *I'm O.K., not good, not bad, but O.K.* I knew that she was from Poland and spoke Polish more often than English. Remembering a couple of words in Polish from growing up with immigrant parents, I replied in affirmation, *dubja* (good).

"Oh," she exclaimed, leaning back with surprise, her eyes widening. "You mean you speak Polish!" Those were the only other words I had ever heard her speak until then.

One day I was teaching a class in acupressure for relieving common ailments. Although Fran didn't like to attend activities, always preferring to stay by herself in her room or in the hallway, she surprised me this time by nodding her head in affirmation. I don't think she knew exactly what acupressure was, but it sparked enough interest for her to want to go.

There were ten elders present, all in wheelchairs. I arranged them in a semi-circle, close enough together so I could go around to show each one where and how to find the acupressure points, as well as have them work with each other on finding points. Fran was her usual quiet self, but when I came to show her one of the points on the hand, her eyes widened in delight. She kicked her leg up into the air, lifted her other arm spreading her fingers wide, as if saying yes to this moment, yes to the delightful pleasure of sensation.

"Oh my, oh my," she exclaimed, moving her head back and forth, smiling in sheer elation, like I had never seen her smile before. Then, she let out a long sigh of relief. "Oh," she exclaimed again, "Oh my, oh my," as if she had been a caged tiger and was now finally freed from her cage. She looked blissful, laughing, then sighing with a slight orgasmic quiver.

"You must like it," I said, still holding the point.

"It's good!" she said. "It's good!"

In that moment, at exactly the same time, every single elder turned their head in her direction, with hands covering their mouths in laughter. No one would have expected Fran to respond like that.

"She likes it!" I said.

"Yes! Yes! Yes! It's good." Fran exclaimed. The laughter rose, as Fran's voice rose higher and higher. "Yes! Yes! Yes!" she cried out.

In all my years of working in skilled nursing, I had never seen anyone express pleasure like that. Meanwhile, at the far end of the semi-circle, my two sweet, soft-spoken lady friends were laughing, slapping their knees, holding their ribs in ribald laughter. I did not have to ask them what they were laughing about: I could tell that it was something *naughty*, but I asked anyway.

With a glimmer of mischief in her eyes, Rosie laughed so hard that tears were rolling down her cheeks as she replied, "We're just wondering if Frank over there could still get it up. What do you think?"

"You two!" I chaffed, while looking over at Frank in his wheelchair smiling quietly, contentedly, and seemingly oblivious to the scene. I noticed that he did not have his hearing aids in and probably could not hear, but my guess was that he sensed something, not only between the two ladies, but the energy stirred in the room by Fran.

The power of touch. Was that what Fran really wanted all that time? To be touched? Was that what all her *hey, hey, heys* meant after all?

It made me realize how powerful touch is. I don't mean the touch that goes on daily when a caregiver dresses and bathes the residents, or when the nurse touches the arm with a needle, but another kind of touch—a touch that is healing, and that holds intention and love. Although the daily routine of the nurse's touch or the caregiver's dressing and bathing can be soothing, more often than not it becomes a mechanical routine that needs to get done quickly because there are many residents waiting. How often are elders in skilled nursing *really* touched?

Wow! I thought. This is wonderful. Fran was moved to laughter and bliss. And I laughed too, delighting in the pleasure of touch shared by everyone in that room in that hour.

Further thoughts

Don't feel hemmed in by your elder's previous interests. Explore and experiment with something new. Don't be afraid to think out of the box.

I once worked with an elder who didn't graduate from high school and who worked in a factory most of her life, in addition to raising a family. She was unhappy most of the time, always complaining, never satisfied, but her whole outlook on life suddenly changed when I brought in a video of the whirling dervishes of Turkey. She was utterly fascinated so I began reading poems to her by the 13th century Sufi mystic, Jelaluddin Rumi. These readings changed her life!

Just as healing touch transformed Fran's life in that moment. These miraculous moments are acts of grace that we can invite into our lives.

Suggestions for creating engaging and inspiring activities

Create more opportunities to cultivate community through the healing arts. Consider offering a workshop by a trained professional in one of the following modalities:

♦ **Basic acupressure techniques for common ailments**. "Acupressure is an ancient healing art that uses the fingers to press key points on the surface to the skin to stimulate the body's natural self-curative abilities. When these points are pressed, they release muscular tension and promote the circulation of blood and the body's life force to aid healing." (Michael Reed Gach, *Acupressure's Potent Points*, p.3)

♦ **Feldenkrais**. Feldenkrais uses gentle movement and directed attention to improve movement and enhance human functioning. These techniques help to increase ease and range of motion and improve flexibility and coordination.

♦ **Aromatherapy.** Aromatherapy uses essential oils and other aromatic plant compounds which are aimed at improving a person's health or mood.

PART V

THE POWER OF STORIES

REMEMBERING LOVE IN FIRST BUD AND BLOSSOM

Essential Points

♦ Provide choices that encourage, invite, and support your elders.
♦ Encourage your elders to reflect on and share their most cherished memories.
♦ Provide opportunities for your elders to experience the healing wonders of nature.

> *Pleasure is the flower that passes; remembrance, the lasting perfume.*
>
> –Jean de Boufflers

Peter became blind in his later years and would sit with his dark glasses on, wearing a gray beret and a wool blanket wrapped around him. Often I found him alone in his room next to the window or in the hallway, confused and disheveled, repeating

149

the same thing over and over again, "I'm cold, I'm cold..." or "Help me, help me ..." or "I gotta go wee wee" or "Where is my wife?"

His kind and very attentive wife lived in assisted living and came twice a day, just before lunch, then again before or after dinner. It saddened Ruth to see Peter like this. Often she remembered the Peter she once knew, and would tell me how wonderful, funny and charming he really is. I knew that to be true, because I saw glimpses—but it was veiled by so many external and internal conditions of being in skilled nursing. Beneath the surface, he *still* was all those things. It just required some digging.

Ruth wanted Peter to be more involved, but he did not like attending most activities unless someone accompanied him who could give him full attention. If he was left alone in a large group, he could not sit still and would begin his cries of, "Where's my wife" or "Help me" or "I'm cold, I'm cold." Some thought it was his inability to concentrate, but I never thought that. Large groups did not work well for him. They were distractions to him, which only irritated him. He needed to be engaged with one other person who could connect to him on another level, and talk about things that mattered to *him*.

When I sat with him quietly reading a story, he became enthralled and would lean over the arm of his wheelchair while listening intently, often sharing a thought-provoking comment or two. Sometimes I would take him outside into the garden. His grip would loosen on the blanket, and the tension in his face would melt into a smile. He enjoyed the sun, the fresh air, and listening to the sound of water rolling gently out of the stone fountain.

"Do you like the sound, Peter?" I asked one day.

"Yes, I like the sound," he replied matter-of-factly, gazing straight ahead. "It brings back memories of growing up."

"How so, Peter?"

"The whooshing sound of the water reminds me of the river in my hometown."

"What was the river like?" I asked.

"It was a river not far from the Jersey shore. You know what the shore is?" he asked in a playful tone of voice, smiling with a dimple piercing through his whiskery cheek.

"Of course I know what the shore is! I'm from New Jersey."

"You're a Jersey girl!" he exclaimed throwing his hands into the air. "The way to my heart! But don't tell my wife that!" he said jokingly while laughing wholeheartedly. His laugh was infectious and made me laugh, too, as our laughter mingled with the sound of the splashing water.

He recalled his boyhood. "You know, we didn't have television like you have today, so the kids would go to the river. That was how we entertained ourselves in those days. We'd fish, sing songs, and swim. Nearby was a field where we'd play baseball. Then in the winter the river froze over, and we'd go ice skating. Then when we got older it was no longer the river, but the shore."

He leaned towards me, and covered his mouth, as if telling me a secret, "The shore was where we would take the girls. But don't tell my wife," he chuckled. "But you know, it took me 40 years to meet my wife. When I found Ruth, that was it for me!" Peter enjoyed talking about his past and telling me humorous stories about his work as a house painter. I enjoyed laughing with him, but I especially loved watching the transformation that came over him. Light and joy flowed from his spirit, animating his whole being. Filled with aliveness, he suddenly became lucid and clear as he remembered.

Sometimes I would give him a rose to smell or lead his hand to the velvety softness of its petals. "Do know what flower it is?" I asked.

"Rose," he replied, breathing in the fragrance again and again, like someone who hadn't had the pleasure of scent in a long time and, like someone who had forgotten what it was like to breathe this deeply. Scents enliven. They open up imagination and memory. "I like it," he said, not wanting to let go of the rose.

One day, his wife came out to join us. When she saw how engaged and voluble Peter was, it not only made her happy, but also playful and flirtatious. She saw what she remembered most of all about him: his humor, and playfulness, and she became like the young woman falling in love with Peter for the first time.

Affectionately taking his arm and kissing him several times on the cheek, she said with a coy smile, "Tell her the story, sweetheart, of how we met."

I could tell he was charmed by her affectionate gesture. "Well, you see, over 50 years ago, when I first moved to California, I looked up a cousin of mine and sent a card with an invitation to dinner, letting him know that I was coming to California, but without realizing it, I wrote the wrong address down. It was supposed to be 58 Mark's Lane. I put 85 Mark's Lane instead. Then I showed up a week later with a box of chocolates in my hand, except it wasn't my cousin or his wife who answered the door, it was Ruth!"

Ruth stroked his shoulder, then leaned over his wheelchair and threw her arms around him and said, "Oh, give me a little kiss, darling!" He smiled, turning towards her. She kissed his cheek, then turned toward me and said, "I was living with my sister at the time. I'll never forget the minute I set eyes on him. I knew he was the one. What a wonderful mistake it was. Wasn't it, darling?" She kissed him again on the cheek. Peter was beaming, thrilled by her amorous behavior. "Fated from the beginning," she continued. "We were meant to be together."

How happy they were sitting in the rose garden by the fountain. Moments like these inspire me to do this kind of work—to experience the joy of others who had forgotten joy, to find out what stirs their hearts.

Peter became a different man when he was deeply engaged. When he was not, he looked like an old, lost soul, confused and disheveled in his wheelchair, with his pants unzipped and his diaper sticking out, shouting, "I got a go wee, wee, I got a go wee, wee" or "I'm cold, I'm cold." Perhaps he wasn't really cold at all, but he had the need for human connection and the warmth that stirs memories of childhood days and the beginnings of love in first bud and blossom.

Further thoughts

Falling in love is always a favorite theme to reflect on, a sure way to bring much delight and lively conversation.

Suggestions for creating engaging and inspiring activities

For family caregivers:

◆ Does your loved one still keep that special box of cards, love letters, pressed flowers or leaves from the first kiss or date? If so, encourage him or her to go through and share (if comfortable doing so).

◆ If you have pictures or videos, dig them out of the closet and view together. Encourage mom or dad to share stories. This can become a most endearing and memorable event for you as caregiver. You may well hear stories you never heard before that expand your understanding of your loved ones, and what their life was like before you came into the picture. If there were special meals or desserts that were shared between your parents, try recreating that special dessert or meal— tastes and smells bring back memories marvelously!

◆ Was there a particular place associated with falling in love, or with the first date, that is easy to get to? If so, take your loved ones there.

STORY MAGIC

Essential points

- Inspire your elders by reading more stories and poems aloud.
- Bring comfort, joy, humor, peace, and healing through stories.
- Create community through storytelling.

> *A story is like water*
> *that you heat for your bath.*
> *It takes messages between the fire*
> *and your skin. It lets them meet,*
> *and it cleans you …*
> *Water, stories, the body…*
> *all the things we do, are mediums*
> *that hide and show what's hidden.*
>
> Rumi, Story Water

I love stories. There is something magical held within them. Another world opens up, rekindling a sense of wonder and awe, giving us a glimpse of something other than *this:* this world with its everyday problems, worries and concerns, its physical ailments and discomforts that elders suffer day in and day out. Stories can take us to the highest realm of our being as we step away from *this place*, and enter that *other* place.

Stories can heal and transform. Stories are the one place I know I can go to when I am sad or lonely, and somehow the sadness diminishes, at least momentarily, while I ponder some eternal truth or mystery, some hidden gem. I keep a collection of stories. Each one has been carefully selected. They have been gathered from different sources from around the world with many from India. Others are from the Jewish mystical tradition and are known as Hasidic tales. Sometimes friends send me stories by unknown authors or from unknown sources.

I love telling stories, bringing the story to life, so that each person can *see*. My hope is to stir a sense of magic within each elder, giving them something to ponder, something that ignites the soul. But, of course, it doesn't always happen like that. Some fall asleep. Some are restless and bored. But there are always a few who listen, who are moved in some way. Sometimes when I try to open up discussion, the elders have much they want to talk about. Other times there are no words except for a "Wow," or a "That was beautiful," or "Thank you for bringing us this story."

Quite often Sandra would exclaim, "I have never heard stories like these in my life. They are meaningful and make me think about other things beside *this*. They take me away from all my problems." I was especially happy to hear this because Sandra became agitated very quickly and was always calling for attention and assistance, whether she really needed it or not. She also became bored easily. Rarely could she sit in silence, yet each time I read, she listened intently with a sense of wonder. Not once did she call or yell for someone to come and help her, so in the present moment was she. Nothing else distracted her.

Gloria, still quite lucid, highlighted in her monthly calendar the storytelling hour with an asterisk. She was always the first to come. Ordinarily, she did not attend activities. She spent much of her time reading or in Independent Living. When a week passed and I did not read, she would remind me to please read again. "We need more of this," she would say.

Emma, who had Alzheimer's and was not able to focus for very long, would not only listen, but then would clap whole-heartedly and exclaim, "Oh! That was marvelous, simply marvelous!"

Dory would follow Emma in clapping and say, "We need stories! Bring more!" Jill was not able to speak or walk, and typically cried and fumbled with an agitated motion, yet when listening to stories, she became calm. Her eyes even held a bit of a sparkle. Something in her expression made me realize she was *seeing* the story come alive, although she could not express it, but her silence and equanimity spoke of an inner truth beyond words.

And there was Bee, her eyes and mouth open wide with the word "Wow." Often she would start to say something, gesticulating as if to convey the words and thoughts that were bursting within her. Part of a sentence would come, but the words completing the sentence were lost. Yet it did not matter. What was important was that she was touched deeply inside her soul, a *big wow* flowing within her.

One day, I was amazed to discover that Shelia, who was always snoozing, was in fact listening to every single word. When I finished, her head suddenly popped up, her eyes flashing open as she said, "Aah, that was really beautiful. Tell us another one."

Suggestions for creating engaging and inspiring activities

♦ **Facilitate a weekly storytelling hour.** Bring your own favorite stories to read aloud and invite the elders to share theirs. For a list of books I've used that the elders

have enjoyed, please see the suggested reading and
resource list in the appendix.

♦ **Storytelling for a group.** Invite your elders to sit in
a circle. Ask them to choose the story theme. You can
also use a picture or series of pictures to help inspire the
story. One elder speaks the first sentence, then another
speaks the second, etc. until they have finished the story.
It is a good idea to record the story, then transcribe it
onto paper.

♦ **Bookmaking as an individual or group activity.** Put
together in book form the story the elders created along
with pictures, drawings, and anything else that feels
appropriate for the subject matter. Be as creative as you
like with designing the book, and use ribbon or anything else appealing that will hold the book together.
Card stock works well and comes in a wide variety of
colors.

BENJAMIN'S SHOES
AND
A TALE FROM THE BAAL SHEM TOV

Essential points

♦ Research each elder's history thoroughly and design activities accordingly.
♦ Think out of the box.
♦ Bring inspiration, joy, peace, and healing through reading stories and poems aloud.
♦ Be a source of comfort and support.
♦ Aspire to be a channel for love.

> *The best portion of a good man's life — his little, nameless, unremembered acts of kindness and love.*
>
> —William Wordsworth

Benjamin sat upright in his easy chair, with his plump hands folded in his lap, alert to every sound, syllable, and nuance, eager not to miss a word of the story I was reading to him.

Long ago, there lived a cobbler with his wife, Rivka, and their eight children. They were so poor that they were barely able to clothe and feed their children, let alone to pay their rent. Months had passed, and one day while Rivka was away at the market, the landlord came with the police and hauled the cobbler and their children away to sell them into slavery.

When Rivka returned, her neighbor came to tell her what she had witnessed. Rivka was shocked, as she stood in a now empty house. Everything was gone — most importantly, her family. Not knowing what else to do, she went to the landlord and begged and pleaded, but the landlord sent her away without a thought. But then suddenly the landlord had an idea: if he asked twice as much as he could get from the slave market, he would be a rich man. An impossible task, he thought, but he had nothing to lose, so he called her back and agreed to ransom them back if she paid him ten thousand rubles. She could not believe the amount he was asking. Ten thousand rubles! A hundred rubles would have been hard enough to come up with, but ten thousand! Where could she possibly get ten thousand rubles? It seemed impossible.

Despondent, she left the landlord wondering how she would ever come up with the money. She reached into her pocket and pulled out three rubles. That was all she had. There was nothing she could do. She had given up all hope.

As she was walking ponderously along the dirt path leading back home, a terrifying thought came to her. What would happen if her children were separated from her husband? What if her husband ended up alone? What would happen if he became sick? He was old. Or what if he was not fed and starved to death? What if he died and was alone? What would happen to him? Where would he be buried? She would not even know where he was or when to say Kaddish [a special Jewish prayer said for the soul of the deceased].

And if his children were not there to say Kaddish, who would say Kaddish for him? Who? There would be no one…

As she continued walking, she saw a beggar and gave the beggar one ruble and said to him, "Please say Kaddish for my husband." After telling the beggar her husband's name, she continued walking home, when another thought came to her. What about all the people who die, who have no one in the world to say Kaddish for them? What about all those people? So saddened was she, when she thought about all the people in the world who have no homes, no families, and no one to say Kaddish for them, that she turned around and walked back to the beggar and gave him another ruble and said, "Please say Kaddish for all the people who have no one to say Kaddish for them, please pray for all those forgotten souls."

As she walked away, another thought came to her, and she went back again to the beggar, who held the two rubles in his hands. She still had one more left and gave it to him and said, "When you pray for all those forgotten souls, pray with your whole heart and soul, give everything to those prayers." But this time, Rivka did not walk away. Instead she sat in the fields nearby listening to his prayers, and did he pray! With a broken heart he prayed, and she began to weep because she heard how hard he prayed and much he put his whole heart and soul into it, just like she had asked. She felt the power of those prayers and kept weeping as the sun set.

Hours passed, and when he was finished, she began walking home. Suddenly a beautiful golden carriage with four horses appeared on the road. This was very strange, she thought. She had never seen a carriage like this before, and certainly never on this dirt path, but what was even stranger was that the carriage stopped near her. Inside was a well-dressed gentleman asking her for directions. Then he asked her if she wanted a ride. At first she said no. After all, he was a stranger, but he insisted, and when she saw how sincere and harmless he seemed, she accepted his kind offer…

* * *

Pausing, I looked at Benjamin, who was now reclining, with his eyes closed and his head propped back. I closed the book and was about to leave when he opened his eyes behind his thick glasses, propped his head up and said, "But you didn't finish. What happens in the carriage?" Promptly, I sat down and continued…

The gentleman asked her many questions, and before Rivka knew it, she was telling him the entire story of her family and the plight she was in. She also told him about her fears of her husband dying alone, and how she gave the beggar her last few rubles to say Kaddish, not only for her husband, but for all the poor people who die without having anyone to pray for them. When the carriage arrived at her doorstep, just as she was about to get out, something happened that was so miraculous. He wrote a check out for ten thousand rubles. She could not believe her eyes.

The following day she ran to the bank with the check, but when she handed it to the clerk, he looked at her strangely, excused himself for few minutes, and went away with the check in hand. While waiting nervously, she wondered, was the check real or was it some cruel joke that the gentleman in the carriage was playing on her? When the clerk came back, he was accompanied by his supervisor, who took Rivka by the hand, and led her to his office. "Where did you get this check?" he asked. After she told him the entire story, he pointed to the many portraits on the wall above his desk, and asked if the gentleman in the carriage, who gave her the check, looked like any of the pictures.

She surveyed them all, and without a doubt recognized one as the gentleman. When she told him which one it was, the supervisor turned pale. The check in his hand was written by his father, who died five years earlier. He was the only child and had never said Kaddish.
(story adapted from *God is a Verb,* David A. Cooper, p.273-276)

Benjamin gazed at me, yet not at me but through me, as if pondering the story and the soul within the storyteller. He smiled warmly as he often did. I wanted to ask what was passing through his mind, but before I could he asked me in his usual quiet way, "Do you believe the story?"

"I believe in the power of prayer. Do you?"

Squinting in a struggle to see, he looked up at a framed picture of his deceased wife on the wall, then turned to me, nodded, and asked, "Will you pray for me when I am gone?"

"But you are still alive, and I pray for you now."

"But when I am gone will you pray for me?"

"You will be here for a long time."

"We can never be certain, not you, not me."

"I will pray for you always with my whole heart and soul."

***

Benjamin loved stories. This was one among many that I read to him. He looked forward to my daily visits and would wait anxiously, listening for the chime of ankle bells, by which he came to recognize me. With his oversized gray pants held up by suspenders, he stood in the doorway of his room anticipating my arrival.

Benjamin was a quiet man who kept to himself. Two months went by without my having met him. I only knew his name because I saw it every day next to a row of unmarked bubbles on the activities attendance sheet. Why have I not met him, and who is he? I wondered. "And *why* doesn't he *ever* come out of his room?" I asked the Activity Director.

"He prefers being alone, and he doesn't seem to have any interest in activities," she replied.

"But he *must* have interests," I responded.

"I heard that he is supposed to be a really smart man."

"Oh, I see."

Benjamin was a mystery to me. Immediately I set out to meet him. I wanted to get to know him, what made him tick, what kinds of things interested him. It did not take me long to discover he was a humble and simple man, soft-spoken, gentle, and perhaps even a little shy. He liked reading and loved stories.

"What kinds of stories do you like?" I asked.

He liked world literature and was especially fond of the classics. Sometimes I would read short passages from his favorite books. He also was deeply spiritual, so some days I would read mystical stories from India or Hasidic tales. And every day, without fail, he would ask me to tell him another story.

Benjamin was disarming, yet often he caught me by surprise by saying something so unexpected that I would have to pause in reflection. His words would alter my perception, make me see something in a new light, from a different angle. Sometimes with his subtle, quiet sense of humor he would say something incredibly funny that seemed to come out of nowhere.

One day, his daughter, Molly, who like me, loved India, told me about her teacher from India who had changed her life completely. Molly brought a copy of her teacher's book, *The Autobiography of a Yogi*, for her father to read. Benjamin was never garrulous, preferring to use his words sparingly, so there was nothing unusual about his silence as he listened to our conversation, moving his head back and forth while looking up at us intently. "You've got to read this book, Dad. Here is my guru," Molly said.

In his soft-spoken manner, Benjamin said, "And *she* is *my* guru," as he reached up for my hand. "Right here is my guru," he said again smiling, swinging my hand lightly back and forth, "I get all my teachings from her."

We looked at each other and laughed.

"You are a funny man, and you make me laugh!" I replied.

Another day, Molly asked him what advice he would give to someone wanting to live a good life. He replied, "Get married and make lots of babies."

On another occasion, I told Benjamin that I was dating a nice Jewish boy (my husband-to-be) and that I had gone to my very first Seder, a festive ceremonial meal recounting the Exodus story from the Bible, encouraging the participants to see themselves as if they were undergoing this spiritual journey from slavery to freedom.

I then added, "But, boy oh boy, are they ever long! It went on for hours past midnight."

"It took the Jews a long time to cross the desert, you know," Benjamin retorted.

Benjamin was a world-renowned scientist and a prolific writer who had taught at one of the more prestigious universities. He could trace his family back to the Baal Shem Tov, the Jewish mystic and founder of the Hasidic movement in the early 18th century, whose stories I had been reading almost every day for over a month, without even knowing I was reading the stories of Benjamin's remarkable ancestor. Not once did he mention or even hint at his roots going back to the Baal Shem Tov.

That was very much a part of who Benjamin was: one of the humblest human beings I have ever met. He never talked about his many accomplishments or about his work as a scientist and how well-known he was in his field.

Fortunately, Molly told me. I was thrilled to learn so much about Benjamin, and asked him why he never said anything.

"Why?" he said. A long, silent pause followed. He was waiting for me to reply. "Why is it so important?" he asked again. "Does it really mean anything?"

Expectantly, he kept looking at me. I did not know what to say. His question made me ponder, does it *really* matter? And what am I responding to? The fact that he was a world- renowned scientist teaching at a prestigious university? Does that really matter? It does, *yet* ... it *really* doesn't. We get attached to our positions, our titles, our possessions, the things we accumulate — yet how important are those things? Are they truly ours? Things change, we grow old, and we must let them go and leave all those things behind that we once thought of as *ours.*

Benjamin was wise. Throughout his life, even in his younger days, he did his work without becoming *attached,* according to Molly. He was already prepared for this final stage in his life. It was as if he had been preparing for it his whole life. So it *is* important, yet it *isn't.*

Perhaps what matters is the awareness that I am human, and as a human, subject to the same vulnerabilities as every other human, such as sickness, old age and death, and that I have done something good in the world. Maybe the important questions are: Have I made a difference? Have I touched others and made their lives better? Have I brought more love and kindness into the world?

Of course, Benjamin is leaving behind a lifetime of scholarship, papers and books, his accomplishments that helped to advance the work in his field, yet there is something else he is leaving behind. It is the Benjamin whom I have come to know. That Benjamin has touched me deeply.

Years have passed, and he still touches my spirit. Whenever I read a tale from the Baal Shem Tov, I think of Benjamin, who I see as an exemplar of his forefather's great teachings. The Bal Shem Tov was known for his simple piety, joy, humility, love and the great respect he had for every human being, no matter what their stature. All that was in Benjamin's blood.

Benjamin was born in Palestine, as he called it, because he came from there prior to 1948. His memory of the country was during a time when Jews and Muslims lived side by side in a friendly, peaceful manner. Goodness and truth were more important to him than religious beliefs. When I asked him what he loved most of all about his departed wife (who was not Jewish), he said, "Her goodness and kindness." I noticed how often he looked up at the framed picture of his beloved hanging on the wall. She had been a nurse, and her essence was kind and humble, like Benjamin's.

When I wasn't reading to Benjamin, I was either taking him outside in his wheelchair to the park, or to the *Wine and Cheese Hour* in Independent Living. Like many other residents in Skilled Nursing, Benjamin especially looked forward to this weekly program, but his reasons were a little bit different from the others. For him, it wasn't because it was a grand and elegant social affair filled with large crowds and old friends. Benjamin was never much of a social butterfly, even in his younger years. Nor was it the music: show tunes from the 1930s, 40s and 50s played loudly on a grand piano. When Benjamin listened to music, it was usually classical music turned very low.

It is true that he loved red wine, a piece of asiago cheese with grapes and a cracker, but he also loved the journey in getting there as we walked arm in arm. His steps were slow and ponderous, but eventually we made it, with his walker held tightly before him. But what he seemed to love most of all was when I would put on his shoes.

Although years have passed, those shoes still stand out so clearly in my mind. They were worn out but sturdy brown leather sandals with a braided pattern across the top. Like his pants and shirts, they fit loosely. They always had crumbs on them or sticky spots, as if juice had spilled on them, so before slipping them on, I would take a damp cloth and wipe them off. Then I would slip them onto his dry, calloused feet.

I believe that Benjamin looked forward to this little gesture, which became our little ritual. There was something endearing about handling this humble man's shoes. When I went into his room and asked, "Are you ready?" He would look down at his feet and with great effort attempt to pick up one of his shoes. Then he looked up at me in an endearing way as if asking me if I could help. Afterwards, I would take his thick black and gray-rimmed glasses, a style popular in the 1950s, wash them with soap and water, dry them and put them back on his face. I could not help but admire and honor the gentle, wise soul behind those glasses. And arm in arm, we would go.

I would get Benjamin a glass of red wine and some cheese. Although I was often busy escorting other residents in wheelchairs and walkers, I always made sure to sit down with him because I knew how he liked my company. I also knew he could be shy. When the program was over and nearing dinner time, I would bring him back to his room and say goodnight.

One Monday I went to Benjamin's room, and he was not waiting at the doorway. Nor was he sitting on his easy chair. His bed was empty, and his shoes were not near the bed, as they usually were. My heart sank to my stomach. I knew what it meant, but it came as a shock.

I did not expect it, nor did anyone else. It is not unusual for most workers in skilled nursing to know when someone is about to leave their body. Sometimes I leave in the evening and know that the following morning someone will be gone. You sense it and even prepare for it emotionally, but with Benjamin it was different. He was relatively healthy, so it really came as a shock to his family, as well as those who worked with him. Peacefully, he died while sleeping.

I grieved his death for a long time. What saddened me most was that I felt as if I never really said goodbye. There were things I would have liked to have said, like how deeply he touched me, and how much I learned from him. *He was my guru.* I would have liked to have thanked him and to have said again, *I will pray for you always with my whole heart and soul.* That evening I went home and prayed. The following evening, I prayed again. And one day passed into the next, with Benjamin remembered in my daily prayers.

At his memorial service, I stood up and said all those unsaid things, and how he was truly one of the humblest human beings I had ever met in my life. When I sat down, one of the caregivers, who was painfully shy, stood up and said, "I have something to say. 'Humble' is the perfect word to describe Benjamin. I always appreciated how he never talked down to anyone. We were all equal in his eyes. He never yelled or said an unkind word. He always spoke with kindness. He *was* one of the humblest men I have ever met too."

Benjamin may have left behind many things, such as his great scholarship, but the Benjamin I knew was the one who brought something else. He touched the soul, many souls, and I will never forget him.

There was one other thing I regret. I had asked his daughter if I could have some small memento of Benjamin. What I really wanted was those shoes, but the words would not come out. They got caught in my throat. I could not ask for her father's worn-out, stained shoes. I felt embarrassed. Instead, I said nothing, and let her decide. She gave me the book, *Autobiography of a Yogi*, but it was those shoes that my heart wanted most of all.

Further thoughts

Benjamin was remembered for many things, but most of all he was remembered for his kindness, a quality he valued highly. Take time to reflect on how you want to be remembered when you are gone. What are your highest values?

Suggestions for creating engaging and inspiring activities

The following are specific to family caregivers but can be adapted easily by anyone who works with or visits elders.

♦ Read your loved one's favorite poems, short stories, myths, or tales. If you don't know what they are, go through his or her books to see if any notes or markings might indicate his or her favorites. If not, try reading some of your favorites.

♦ Make a collage together using personal photos and any other objects that hold special meaning, such as a shell your loved one may have picked up while walking with his or her beloved, dried out leaves or flower petals from their first date, or perhaps a love note, a handkerchief, or ribbon, etc. This also can be an activity for the whole family. Give it a theme if you like, such as "life with dad in the 1940's," "our dreams for the future," or "falling in love." Follow the intuitive flow of your inner voice. Let that be your guide.

PART VI

CONNECTING TO THE PAST

CHAPTER 20

DAVID AND HANNAH

Essential points

- ♦ Honor and celebrate accomplishments.
- ♦ Be a source of comfort and support.
- ♦ See the goodness in what you have, and be grateful.

> *It is a sweet thing, friendship, a dear balm,*
> *a happy and auspicious bird of calm.*
>
> —Shelley

Whenever I saw them they were hand-in-hand. There was a sweetness about them, a certain tenderness as they walked with slow, small steps, in no hurry, still so in love as they were 75 years ago. Every evening, they sat in the dining room at a table set for two, with a half bottle of red wine and a vase of fresh flowers that had intentionally been moved to the side, so that it wouldn't interfere with their seeing each other. I could not help but stop and smile, while admiring them from afar, until one day I walked over to their table, introduced myself, and told them what a beautiful couple they were and how I hoped that when my husband and I grew old, we would still be so in love and attentive to one another as they were.

Immediately, a warm and friendly relationship began. I learned that they had been living in independent living for a little over a year, and that that year marked their 75th wedding anniversary. By chance, they were both born in the same year and village in Eastern Europe, yet they did not meet until 20 years later when they were students at the same college in America. But when they met, they knew instantaneously they were meant to be together.

Sharing a similar fate and history, they had lived parallel lives. They both had lived in concentration camps during the Holocaust, while still in their early adolescence. Because they lacked proper nutrition, their growth had been stunted, and neither one was more than 5'2". David was a medical doctor who was not only well-versed in medicine but in world literature, history, art, music, piano and violin. Hannah was a teacher, gifted artist and poet.

We shared a common interest; poetry and art, and began exchanging books, as well as conversing about poetry and literature. I told them about a book my husband had written *Songs to My Beloved*. I shared with them the story of how my husband had been longing to meet his life companion. He had been alone for a long time and spent many sleepless nights anguished by his loneliness. He prayed that he would meet his beloved, and in the midst of his prayers he had a sudden insight that if he was longing for her, she must also be longing for him. Thus began his practice of writing letter poems to the spirit of his beloved.

Shortly afterwards, we met. A year later he proposed and read the poems he had composed to me at our favorite spot at the sea, near a stream where two white doves were bathing. I loved the poems and encouraged him to publish them. The book was handed out at our wedding.

David and Hannah were taken by the story, so I brought the book for them to read. She gave me a book of her poems as well. Quickly, I became a big fan of hers. We shared a similar sensibility: the romantic spirit, with the yearning heart, and love of solitude and nature, unhampered by the hands of man. Her poetry, as well as her paintings of landscapes — with a tempestuous sea, a garden left abandoned and wild, and a forest of desolated ruins — reflected that spirit.

I enjoyed getting to know both of them more deeply as time passed, but one day I was shocked when I arrived at work to find Hannah alone, frightened, and waiting nervously at the front desk in skilled nursing. I knew things constantly changed, but somehow I thought it wouldn't happen to either of them. They would always be in independent living walking hand-in-hand, or in the dining room at a table set for two. But there she was, my friend Hannah, holding her arms out to me, sighing with relief, exclaiming how happy she was to see me.

"I don't know anyone. Look at all these sad-looking souls!"

I understood how she felt. I have seen it happen many times. Suddenly, she was in skilled nursing with a whole set of unfamiliar faces, in a setting filled with frenzied activity, call lights and medicine carts, echoing shrieks jarring the senses, where *a bunch of old sick people* (as I have once heard someone in her position say of the elders in skilled nursing) were slumped over in wheelchairs, with unpleasant smells greeting you unexpectedly, and *odd-looking folks* wandering around aimlessly, mumbling to themselves.

While I sat with Hannah, one of our Alzheimer's residents approached her. The woman stared vacantly, patting Hannah's head and chattering away nonsensically.

Although I knew this resident was harmless, Hannah did not. It may have been one of the first times she ever encountered someone with Alzheimer's, and so she did not know what to make of it. I thought she was about to scream, but instead she threw her arms in the air, begging me to help her "get out of this place."

"What does she want? Tell her to go away," she yelled, agitatedly shaking her clenched hands.

I had never seen Hannah like that before, yet I understood the intensity of her fear. I asked where David was. She said he would be there soon. I reassured her that I was there for her and would help her in whatever way I could.

I spent the next 45 minutes talking with her about what had happened. She had fallen down and broken her hip. I sensed there was a decline in her mental condition. The change seemed to occur overnight. I had never known her to be this confused and disoriented. Of course, it could have been the confusion of coming into skilled nursing, but something in me told me that it was more than that.

She was suffering from dementia. I consoled her as best as I could, while introducing her to other residents and staff, so that she wouldn't feel so alone. I hugged her and held her hand until David arrived. From that moment on, he was always with her, except when he had a doctor's appointment or urgent business, or when he returned in the evenings to their apartment in independent living. He would have stayed with her, but it wasn't permitted.

I was grateful I was able to be there for her, as someone who had gotten to know her *before*, while she was still in independent living. I am equally grateful to have been there for many others, who like Hannah, came into skilled nursing frightened and alone. One familiar face can make all the difference in the world.

Unfortunately, Hannah declined quickly. When David was not there, especially in the evenings, she would ask several times where he was and where she was. She had forgotten she was in skilled nursing, as well as why she was there. It was a comfort for her to see me. Although she may not have known how or where she knew me, she remembered I was someone she knew. I was connected with *before all this,* somewhere in her past when things were different, more solid and lucid.

It saddened me to see her that way. I knew she would not recover and that we would soon lose her. Yet I also knew that she had lived an extraordinary life. She had loved the man of her dreams. Together they had shared 75 full, rich years. She had learned and grown. As an artist, she created many inspired and inspiring works. She taught and touched many hearts and minds with her thoughts, ideas, and spirit. She saw the world and raised children.

David saddened me most of all because I knew the transition would be difficult for him. I knew how hard it was for him to see his beloved wife like this, yet he had been preparing and was grateful, always remembering that their lives had been blessed. One day when I asked how he was he said, "I am thankful that we had so many beautiful years together."

Still, I could sense great sadness and emptiness within him. I wanted to do something special for them by honoring Hannah as a poet. I asked her and David if I could organize a program around her poetry. They were enthusiastic. And although she was not feeling up to reading and her eyesight was failing, she asked me if I would read the poems for her.

It was a pleasure to see the old Hannah return during that hour. Joy was in her eyes, which just the day before looked deeply sad and lost. She began talking about her poetry, and was completely lucid. She spoke about the yearning spirit, her love of nature and solitude and how these had always been themes in her work. I asked her questions about her work. She responded eloquently, confidently, qualities recently lost but rediscovered in that hour.

I could see that not only was she proud, but David was proud as well. I could see in her eyes that she was reliving memories of being a young woman in love, creative and passionate: the artist who sat in the forest by a stream, expressing her thoughts through the beauty of words, as her life with David was just beginning.

Hannah continued to decline and grow more disoriented and confused. In less than a month, she passed away, but there was that one hour of reliving past memories, of forgetting an ailing body and mind, where lucidity and joy reigned.

Further thoughts

Although nothing could take away from the grief that David experienced after Hannah died, he always remembered to be grateful for what he did have, and that helped him immensely.

Gratitude uplifts, and helps take us out of our own suffering.

Give thanks in your heart, and share your gratitude with your family, your elders, and your friends.

Suggestions for creating engaging and inspiring activities

♦ Organize a weekly or daily gratitude circle. No matter how difficult life can be, there is always something to be grateful for. Ask your elders to think about the many things for which they are grateful. The more they discover, the more they realize just how many things for which they are grateful!

♦ Invite your elders to make a daily practice of being grateful for at least one thing—such as the roses blooming outside, or their family and all the nice things they do. Encourage them to keep a notebook devoted to gratitude practice, or record it.

♦ Facilitate a card-making activity with precut colored stock paper (comes in a variety of colors and is available at most local arts and crafts stores). Use writing or drawing utensils of each elder's choice. Magic markers, crayons, tempera markers, glitter markers, and colored pencils all work well. Invite your elders to make cards expressing thankfulness to those they are grateful for.

WONDERFUL THINGS COME UNEXPECTEDLY AFTER THE FALL

Essential points

- ♦ Blessings come to those who mourn.
- ♦ Miracles abound everywhere—be open to seeing them.
- ♦ Love never ceases.

> *Don't grieve. Anything you lose comes round in another form.*
>
> Rumi

"Oy, oy, oy," Harry cried out in lament, every day, several times, his eyes like a sad puppy's behind his wire-rimmed glasses, his brows furrowed. His wife, wearing bright red lipstick and a strawberry blond bouffant wig, would sit next to him in her fire engine red electric wheelchair glaring through her thick, plastic-framed glasses.

"Oh, be quiet, Harry," she would say in her husky voice.

"Why do you have to be so mean to me?" he would ask.

"I'm not mean to you," was her reply. Sara was really not mean. This was simply a part of their relationship. She adored Harry, and he adored her. At one time, Harry was the domineering one in the household. Now the roles were reversed, with Harry in his manual wheelchair slowly following his wife, who zipped along expertly in her electric wheel chair: a woman always on a mission, going somewhere, usually to independent living to visit friends or attend a program.

"Wait for me," Harry pouted and whined, with great effort trying to propel the wheels that just did not move fast enough, or at least not fast enough to keep up with Sara.

Pressing the button that would spin her chair around like a top, she would reply sternly, "No, you stay here, Harry, you don't have to follow me everywhere I go."

"But I do," he would say with the *do* trailing off into a whimper.

"Why?"

"Because I do."

"Well, that's not a good enough reason," she would reply brusquely.

Nearly choked up with tears, he would plead, "What if something happens? Then what will I do?"

"Oh, Harry, stop it, nothing is going to happen. I'll be back in a couple of hours."

Theirs was a deep, heartfelt love that had endured over seven decades, with a festive celebration of their 75th wedding anniversary that year.

Sara was once a nurse. At the beginning of her career, she met Harry in the emergency room of a hospital in upstate New York after he had a major car crash and nearly lost his life. He came in unconscious with a broken leg and arm, a couple of cracked ribs, and a severe head wound. She was his nurse, one of her first patients.

The most wonderful thing came out of that accident: they fell in love. Maybe that was why he recovered remarkably quickly. Of course they never shared their feelings with one another during his hospital stay, but shortly after he left, he sent her chocolates and flowers with a card thanking her for her good care, along with a dinner invitation. She accepted, and their love story began.

Sara's role as a nurse never stopped, even in skilled nursing. Whenever Harry became sick, including during the last days of his life, she was by his side, making sure all his needs were taken care of and that his medications were brought in on time. She was his faithful, loving companion. I adored them both. Whenever I think of them, I remember their comical, yet tender and loving relationship, and I can't help but smile and feel once again how deeply they moved me.

Shortly before Harry died, while I thought he was sleeping, I stood by his bed, stroking his forehead gently and whispered, "I will miss you, Harry." I really was not expecting a reply. I didn't even think he heard me. But he opened his eyes, turned his head toward me, with a tear falling from the corner of one eye, reached for my hand and said, "I will miss you too." I will never forget that moment.

But what I remember most of all about Harry was his cries of *oy, oy, oy*. Whenever Sara was away, he sat by the nurse's station sniveling *oy, oy, oy*, without pause. The nurses were exasperated, yet amused by his *oy*. I was charmed by them. There was something endearing about them, and each time I could not resist going to his side and *oy, oy, oy* back to him, matching his tone.

"You are a darling," he would say, smiling, then reply *oy, oy, oy*, more lightly this time.

"Oy, Oy, Oy," I said again.

"Oy, oy, oy," he replied until our words became a little jingle-like song.

As we sang together, the smiling nurses shook their heads in an *oh no, here they go again, those two*.

"What do you think, Harry, we could start our own special *oy* choir?" I once said. He chuckled while we *oyed* a little longer.

* * *

When Harry passed away, it was trying for Sara. They had shared that room for over five years, and with the exception of his recent stay in the hospital, Harry and Sara had never been separated. His presence was felt in every corner, in all his wonderful black and white photographs of mountains, oceans, and forests paths, as well as family photographs, wedding pictures, and their most recent photos of their 75th anniversary.

The most difficult thing for Sara was that his side of the bed was now empty. Every death brings that shock of *how could this be, how could this be?* Harry's death did not seem real. It was as if Harry was still there in that emptiness.

As Sara came to terms with the fact that Harry would not return, she became very lonely and depressed. She no longer zipped around to independent living in her electric wheelchair, and her social life ceased all together. Friends came to visit her, but she stayed in bed most of the day, never feeling quite well enough to get up. Rarely did she eat in the dining room, so her meals were brought to her room.

I went to visit her every day. Most of the time, she was sleeping, and when she was awake, she did not seem the woman I had known before. She expressed painful loneliness and felt as if her life had become meaningless and empty.

Sara's health declined as well, but a few months later, it was as if Harry's presence was still there, not only in the things he left behind, but also in a new bright, shining light that filled her room and brought blessings that she would continue to stay happy and well, until it was her time to go.

She decided to have a roommate. Wondrously, her new roommate was a long-lost, beloved friend from childhood who also had recently lost her husband.

In their reunion, they shared their grief. Quickly, they bonded, becoming inseparable, with Sara never wanting to go to an activity without Ruth. Their room was filled with mirth and laughter. Often they joked with each other about getting married. They both felt blessed that they could be there for one another, creating something new and wonderful!

PART VII

IN THE SPIRIT OF INSPIRATION

SPARKS OF INSPIRATION

Essential points

- Bring more beauty into your elders' lives.
- Provide opportunities for them to experience the healing wonders of nature.
- Seek to inspire; inspiration sparks life.

> *There is something infintely healing in the refrains of nature—the assurance that dawn comes after night, and the spring after winter.*
>
> Rachel Carson, *Silent Spring*

> *Oh, there is a blessing in this gentle breeze,*
> *A visitant that while it fans my cheek*
> *Doth seem half-conscious of the joy it brings*
> *From the green fields, and from yon azure sky. . .*
> *I look about: and should the chosen guide*
> *Be nothing better than a wandering cloud,*
> *I cannot miss my way. I breathe again!*

Traces of thought and mountings of the mind
Come fast upon me: it is shaken off. . .
The heavy weight of many a weary day
Not mine, and such as were not made for me.
—William Wordsworth
The Prelude; or Growth of a Poet's Mind

I am quite sure that Muriel was inspired many times in her life. She was a poet and writer, a scholar and one of the first women ever appointed a dean at her Ivy League school. Quite the rebel in her day, she wore a flapper dress at her wedding to assert her fierce independence during a time when women were little more than objects, meant to be no more than mothers and homemakers.

Tiny and frail, she often raced through the hallway in her wheelchair with clenched fists, ranting and raving at the top of her lungs in her raspy, muciferous voice, as if she were a caged animal who at any moment would go crazy if she were not released. Other times, she sat with her head held down between her hands, as if she had lost all hope and had given up on life. During those moments, I embraced her and said, "I adore you Muriel. Remember that you are my hero." She often lifted her head, mumbled some inarticulate words, smiled affectionately, and took my face between her hands.

During her moments of rage, I tried to understand what was bothering her. She responded to my questions with motions and gestures, using inarticulate half phrases with words that slurred into each other. Often she got frustrated, knowing she was not able to just come out and express it. In exasperation she pressed her hand into her forehead, and shook her head. Then, she would get angry all over again, throw her arms in the air, shake them out of utter frustration, and push me away.

I kept reminding her that I wanted to help her. When I got frustrated with my inability to reach her, I reminded myself that often her anger was connected to physical discomforts, such as a urinary tract infection, which is a common and painful problem in skilled nursing.

By the time I met Muriel, she had lost a lot of her memory and speech. I never got to know her when she still *was* the articulate poet, scholar, and brazen rebel, who had to assert herself in the world of men to make sure she got her rightful position of power and prestige. Fortunately, I learned about Muriel's life from other residents who knew her when she was still in independent living and from a young woman visitor whom Muriel had befriended years before at her church congregation.

After several falls, Muriel was transferred, without much choice, to skilled nursing. Severely debilitated, she could no longer walk, something she once greatly enjoyed. She also had dementia and severe depression, but sparks burned through her depression, at least momentarily.

My aim was to find those sparks. Knowing Muriel's love of poetry, I started a poetry circle, hoping she would come, but each time I invited her, she declined, so I stopped asking. The circle continued with great success with a regular group of about seven to ten faithful attendees.

One week while I was in the middle of reading the Wordsworth poem quoted at the beginning of this chapter, Muriel strolled in. Instead of being in her typical anxious, aimless wandering state, she clearly not only *heard* the words, but she was inspired and came to hear more.

It was as if the words were calling her, speaking to her in some deep way. Determined, her deceptively frail, tiny arms became strong and feisty as she propelled her wheelchair through the door with a clear intention to get where she wanted to go, no matter what. Quickly she got herself to her preferred place: the table where I sat with a stack of books.

Expertly, she turned the wheelchair to sit right next to me. With her hands held in her lap, she listened intently, her eyes sparkling. When I finished, she smiled, clapped her hands, nodded in approval and said, "Very good."

"Wow," I exclaimed, "How happy I am that it meets your approval, Dr. Brown." She sat focused in the same spot for the rest of the reading. She even had an expression of awe and wonder, which I hadn't seen before. Perhaps the poems evoked memories of her past life, the days of rebelliousness coupled with inspiration and great devotion. After the reading, she picked up the books, silently surveying their contents. She took her time perusing the pages, saying nothing, only nodding and smiling in approval of my collection.

I read to her many times after that. Her response depended on her constantly fluctuating mood. If the poetry did not touch her, I tried shifting her mood by giving her a hand massage.

One day while massaging her hand with the calloused bump on her third finger, I told her how special her hands were. "These hands," I declared, "paved the way for a generation of women to follow. They are the hands of my hero! And that little bump belongs to none other than a writer and scholar. Don't you forget that!"

She chuckled.

Something else, I discovered, could shift Ruth's mood dramatically, instantaneously. One day when she was in a highly agitated mood, I tried everything to calm her, but to no avail, until I asked if she wanted to go outside for a stroll in the park. She nodded "yes."

I did not realize then that she loved nature. Her whole life had been spent outdoors. Nature inspired her, but when she came to skilled nursing, all that was suddenly taken away from her.

How depressing it must be to never see that world and always be cooped up inside, wandering hallways and corridors and rooms that are sterile with noisy, artificial lighting! She loved forests with their smells of eucalyptus and pine mixed with damp earth and the sea with its tumultuous lapping of waves against shore. She loved gardens, plants, flowers, birds, and trees, and once, she could name each one.

It did not take me long to see that nature was exactly what she needed to brighten her spirit.

The moment we stepped outside, Muriel responded to the sun and slight breeze. She held up her hands, palms open, looking up into the sky as if to give praise and thanks for the beauty of the day. Her usual agitated expression shifted to openness and wonder. She was alive again and inspired.

When we passed a red hibiscus bush, she asked me to stop. She reached over and lifted the flower up to her nose. Closing her eyes, she swept the soft petals across her cheek. I plucked one for her, which she held as if it were a precious jewel, while we continued our journey. When we passed a bush of blooming jasmine, she pointed, letting me know she wanted to stop there as well. While reaching over to smell its luscious fragrance, she smiled and articulated the word *beautiful.* Sparks of delight animated her eyes.

"You let me know whenever you are ready," I said and let her lead the way. She motioned when she was ready, pointing to the park across the street, with its grassy landscape and towering oaks, its paths winding around a lake with ducks and geese. We stopped to look at them, and I could tell by her motioning hands that she would have liked to feed them. Holding her hands up again, she looked up, as light and shadow from the oak trees moved gently across her face, like a god touching her with its eternal mystery. It was as if she had words that wanted to pour forth in poetic expression, but instead held them within as a feeling of *yes, this is the world, this is nature, and you and I are alive.*

That day I saw Muriel truly come alive. She seemed to be more lucid and her speech was clearer, more coherent. From that day forward, a stroll outside became a part of our regular routine. Whenever she was in one of those moods, the nurses would say, "She needs you. You know what to do."

The first year I met Muriel, I asked her on Valentine's Day if she would be my Valentine, but I knew I was being much too silly for the Ivy League professor and dean. "I will bring you chocolates and flowers. Please, oh please, be my Valentine."

"Don't be so silly," she said, waving me away.

"But you are my darling and my hero!" I replied.

A slight smile appeared, yet still she shooed me away again. But the following year, after we had experienced many inspired moments in the park, I asked her again if she would be my Valentine. This time, she quickly replied, "Of course, I will be your Valentine. You are my darling too." She patted my cheeks with her bony little hands.

"How happy I am!" I exclaimed. Finally, the rebel had relented.

Further thoughts

Nature is a healing balm. It helps to ground and connect us. It helps bring peace and solace, clear the mind, and provide the space where our deep inner voice can be heard. Let nature nurture you. Take advantage of its bounty, beauty, and blessing.

Suggestions for creating inspiring and engaging activities

♦ Take your elders to the park, lake, or some other natural setting.

♦ Spend time with your elders silently observing the life around you — birds flitting about, squirrels at play, flowers blooming and trees sprouting and shedding leaves, the formation of the leaves. If you see a pretty flower, point it out, touch and smell it. Use all your senses!

♦ If you see a beautiful leaf or rock, pick it up. Invite your elders to make up a story together about the life of this object, where it might have come from, how it got to be where it is, and what message, advice, or words of wisdom the object has to share with each person today. If someone has a concern or worry, ask what the object tells him or her to do.

♦ Set up a bird feeder or bird bath outside.

♦ Create a butterfly garden.

♦ Bring in a small water fountain. The sound of water is soothing.

♦ If you live in the city where it might be difficult to go out into nature, create an aviary or a small garden with plants and herbs. Watch things grow; measure their growth to witness the process. If your elders choose to grow herbs, provide some of the harvest to the chef of the community to be used in preparing resident meals.

♦ Use CD's with nature sounds and/or watch nature shows.

THE STORY OF IRIS

Essential points

♦ Foster creativity.
♦ Encourage self-expression.

> *A Sensitive Plant in a garden grew,*
> *And the young winds fed it with silver dew,*
> *And it opened its fan-like leaves to the light,*
> *And closed them beneath the kisses of Night.*
>
> *And the Spring arose on the garden fair,*
> *Like the spirit of Love felt everywhere;*
> *And each flower and herb on Earth's dark breast*
> *Rose from the dreams of its wintry rest."*
>
> —Percy Bysshe Shelley,
> *The Sensitive Plant*

Iris, soft-spoken, even tempered, and relatively young at 75, with barely a wrinkle on her cherubic face, was one of the first elders I served. I facilitated a small group for those who wanted to write poetry. Many could not write because of arthritis; others had very poor eyesight, so I was there to help get the poem on the page.

The group did not last long. Many could not focus for very long and lost interest, but Iris seemed to be particularly responsive to words, their beauty and expression. Soon it became clear that she had a real interest in poetry. She had never written any poems, but always wanted to. Yet like many adults, she felt that she could not write, was not creative and would never be good enough.

The truth is that we all can write or be creative in some way. We just have to change the way we think about writing and creativity. Masters take years to develop, but we don't have to be masters. We can choose from so many different forms: painting, making a piece of pottery or jewelry, weaving, writing a poem, etc.

Writing can be a way of uncovering and expressing our deepest longings. And so it was with Iris. She just needed someone to help birth her inspiration, so I became her midwife. She led the way, while I transcribed for her.

One day, I came to work and did not see her in the group. When I asked about her, I was told she was not feeling well, so I went to her room immediately. She lay propped up in bed. This was unusual. She was always up, dressed and ready to go. Her cheeks were a bit pale, but she still seemed to be doing well, just not well enough to get out of bed. When she saw me, she was happy and said how sorry she was that she was not able to come to the group.

"I kept thinking about what I was missing," she said.

"Do you feel up to writing today?" I asked.

"Well, I really want to ..." she replied, looking at the wall near the side of her bed, "but, you know I'm not very good."

Turning toward me again, she continued, "You know that I am not a poet and I can't really write."

Although her words reiterated what she and many of us were oddly taught to believe, her heart spoke her true wish to write poetry.

Pressing my hand to her hands, interlocked and resting on the sheet over her chest, I said, "But you can. It's not that you can't write. It's that you *think* you can't write."

"But I don't know the first thing about rhyming and formal structure. You know that."

"And *you know* what I always say about that. Forget about it! It only hinders and intimidates. Throw away the idea of having to stick to a traditional form with its rhyme schemes and cadences. Don't think so much about how you think a poem should be written. Think of it more like your own personal expression, like an exercise. Let what wants to come out, out. It is like setting free what has been locked within a cage."

Iris pondered. She slipped her hand out from beneath mine, and affectionately placed it on top of mine.

"I brought the poem you started with me," I said. "It's a beautiful beginning. You just need to finish. Do you feel up to it today?"

While working with Iris in the group, I noticed that she mentioned her name often, as if it held some deep significance for her, so I asked her to tell me more about what her name meant to her. I wrote down the words she dictated — her mother, the love she had for her mother, her mother's garden, and how she loved irises.

Then I read her words to her. Intently, she listened. She seemed to be awakening to some beautiful discovery. The expression on her face revealed no worries, no cares, only love and joy. She was remembering other days of sunlight and flowers.

"Tell me more about your mother," I asked.

She replied exuberantly, "My mother loved irises. It was her favorite flower. She grew all kinds of flowers, trees and vegetables, but because she was so fond of irises, they grew everywhere. Shortly after she and my father moved into the little white house with her big beautiful garden, she became pregnant with me. She told me that one day in spring before I was born, warm winds came that were soft, gentle, and fragrant. As she felt them against her face and hair, it seemed to her that those winds were telling her that the baby inside should be called Iris. So my mother named me Iris.

"How she loved that garden! How I loved it, too! When I think of the garden, I think of my mother. It was her haven, her place of retreat, because my father was so demanding. He always expected so much from her. She didn't work outside the house, but she worked harder and more than he did, raising four children, doing all the cooking and cleaning. It made me sad, because when I grew older I saw how hard it was on her, yet the garden brought her peace. It became a place she could call her own, where she found quiet time, where she was able to collect a part of herself, which was lost during the chores of the day and the demands of my father.

"My mother's gentle beauty was reflected in her garden. She painted with flowers and trees like an artist paints with color on canvas."

"Wow," I said, "that's a beautiful way to phrase it – painted with flowers and trees like an artist paints with color on canvas. What do you mean you're not a poet?"

She smiled. "What was the garden like?" I asked. "Tell me what it looks like, how it tastes and smells."

"I remember spring most of all. I helped my mother plant. I remember baby red robins chirping in nests in our maple trees. Sometimes it rained, a nice warm rain. One day I saw a rainbow for the first time. It was so beautiful. I pointed it out to my mother, and she told me that my name, her favorite flower, Iris, was also another name for a rainbow, so I was like a flower and a rainbow to her. I must have brightened her days."

She paused, her eyes gleaming, while basking in the memory. Like her good scribe, I kept writing. "What did you write so far?" she asked. I read her words and asked how she wanted to begin.

After some thought, she replied, "When I think of my mother, I think of our garden…"

She paused and grew frustrated. I asked her more questions. Is this what you mean? Or is this what you mean? Do you like this word? Or do you like that word or phrase better? At times, when she was stuck, I offered suggestions from the original group of ideas. And I wrote them down, line by line.

We were just beginning. There was so much more I wanted to know. I wanted to hear her describe her mother and the affection they had for one another, but her eyes were closing. She was tired, and I whispered, "You rest. I'll come back tomorrow. We'll finish then." In a moment of wakefulness, she opened her eyes and asked me to read what I had written. So I read the rough draft to her:

When I think of my mother,
I think of our garden
that she so loved,
that I loved, too.

My mother's gentle beauty was reflected in the garden
as she painted
with flowers and trees like an artist
paints with colors on canvass.

The garden was her haven;
a place of retreat
away from the endless chores
and demands of my father.
Peace was hers in the garden,
where irises grew in abundance,
because they were my mother's favorite flower.

She once told me that when she was pregnant with me
warm fragrant spring winds came
and blew against her face and hair.
They held a message that her baby should be called Iris.
And so I was named.

We planted in the spring,
while birth gave life to red robins
chirping in nests in the maple trees.

Sometimes it rained,
but it was a nice warm rain.
One day a rainbow appeared,
the first one I ever saw.
I pointed it out to my mother.
She said that my name,
her favorite flower, meant rainbow.

I like to think that Iris brightened my mother's days,
just like the irises in the garden did,
just like the springtime did with the warm rain
and the rainbow that followed...

"It's beautiful," she exclaimed, her eyes glistening, but after a
pause said, "but I didn't write it. You did."

"No, Iris. I only helped you. You spoke about your mother
and the garden that you both loved and planted in spring, and
the warm rain and the rainbow. The words came from you. Aren't
they your thoughts? They're not mine. I don't have a beautiful
name like Iris that means rainbow. That is really something! And
it is only you, your thoughts and words."

"It is, isn't it?" she replied.

"If you want to change anything, let me know."

Shaking her head back and forth on the pillow, with her curled hair spread out like the petals of a sunflower, she said, "No, it's beautiful. It is hard to believe it is mine."

"Well, it is."

She became quiet again. Her eyes started to close. I knew it was enough. We did our work for the day. She needed rest.

"It is beautiful, Iris. When I go home tonight, I'll type it and bring it for you tomorrow. " Nodding, she smiled warmly, her sunny spirit shining through — a gentle beauty just like the beauty of her mother. Drifting off into a landscape of dreams with gardens, irises, rainbows, and her dear sweet, mother, she started to fall asleep. Just as I was about to leave, she reached for my hand. With her eyes still closed, as if not wanting to be taken out of her lovely dream, she whispered, "Thank you. Come back tomorrow. I'll be waiting."

I kissed her on the forehead and thanked her for sharing such beautiful memories with me. That evening I typed her poem and printed it on lavender paper in a pretty calligraphy-style font, enlarged and easy to read. The following day, excitedly, I rushed to work, eager to share the poem with her. I could hardly wait to see the expression on her face— this was her first poem, which she believed she could not write.

When I went to her room, her bed was empty, stripped down to reveal the bare air mattress beneath, and her wheelchair was by the side of her bed. My stomach clenched. I knew what it meant.

The charge nurse informed me it had happened yesterday evening. "At least her passing was peaceful," she said. "Iris was not in any pain."

Silently, I said a prayer and recited her poem to her, as if her spirit were still there, and she could still hear. And in my heart I knew she could. She was listening. Suddenly, I felt a wave of peace come over me. It was Iris' peace.

Iris, may your spirit, your name, your mother and her garden with the luminous light of the rainbow always live on.

Suggestions for creating inspiring and engaging activities

♦ Write poems as an individual or group activity:

- Ask the elders if there is a special meaning behind their name, and invite them to write a free form poem about it. Most people have a story to tell about where their name came from.

- Supply a variety of images. Invite each elder to choose one and write a free verse poem about the image chosen.

- Read a short vivid poem aloud, such as *I Wandered Lonely as a Cloud,* by William Wordsworth. Invite your elders to close their eyes while you read the poem slowly. Then ask them to write their own free verse poem, as inspired by the poem. This activity can also be adapted for writing a group poem. One elder begins with the first line, then another writes the next line, etc. until the poem is finished.

- Type one of your favorite poems in a font that is large enough for someone with poor eyesight to see. Print and cut out each word, phrase, or sentence, and arrange them on a table for your elder to choose from. If you are working with a group, put the pieces in a bowl or hat that gets passed around. This activity works best when you begin with a phrase and continue from there. I've seen some pretty amazing poems assembled from many of e.e. cummings' poems, including, *i thank you God for most this amazing day,* and Robert Frost's, *The Road Not Taken.* Please see the suggested reading for books I've enjoyed using.

- Provide three end words for three tercets, and compose a poem. A tercet is a group of three lines of verse, often rhyming.

- Have the elders write a group poem. One person begins with the first line, then the second person continues with the second line, etc. until there are thirty lines and the poem is complete.

PART VIII

SURRENDERING TO THE FLOW OF THE SEASONS

24

ACCEPTANCE AND SURRENDER

Essential points

- Honor your elders' choice for solitude, silence, and introspection.
- Be patient.
- Learn to listen to the same story again and again as if for the first time.
- Be present.
- Provide opportunities to experience the wonders of nature.

> *These roses under my window make no reference to former roses or to better ones; they are for what they are; they exist with God today. There is no time to them. There is simply the rose: it is perfect in every moment of its existence.*
>
> —Emerson

Look at the lilies, how they grow; they neither toil nor spin.

—Matthew 6:28

I visited Marie almost every day. She liked sitting in her room staring through the window at the world outside the glass: the little courtyard with its rose bushes, its pink buds opening wide in the bright sun, wider each day, blossoming, then fading and scattering to the ground, petals left on grass, on pavement. Marie watched the changes and knew each flower intimately, as if they were her own children and she were watching them grow. She could tell you about each one.

Marie told me the same stories again and again. I listened as if for the first time, repeating the same *oohs* and *aahhs*, and *wows*, and *is that so?* She liked telling the stories of her three husbands, especially her last one, because he was the one she loved most. "He liked to have a little drink of bourbon, sometimes one too many at times, but that was O.K.," she would say. "He made up for it in other ways, with so many other wonderful qualities."

She liked telling me stories about her travels around the world, to places like India, Ireland, and Thailand. "How wonderful it is to be alive and free," she often said. I never got the feeling that Marie was depressed about growing old. She seemed to have come to terms with it in a quiet acceptance. In between stories and sentences, she would pause while gazing outside the window, as if she were reliving the past joyously, yet still present to this world with me there sitting on the bed, and the world outside the glass with the rose bushes blossoming and fading, and the hummingbirds humming at the feeder that she herself had placed outside her window.

Marie had forgotten that she told me the same stories every day, and that by now I knew them as intimately as she did. Yet she was generally aware of fading memory. "I'm getting forgetful," she would say, her head bobbing with an aged quiver. "It's what happens, you know, when you grow old," she would say in her voice that was becoming hoarser and wearier as the days passed.

Maybe it wasn't really about being forgetful, but about remembering and the importance of remembering. I let her remember anew, each time, as if she were reliving each moment for the first time, seeing her Joe drinking a little bourbon, sometimes one too many. She would smile with a twinkle in her blue eyes, or sometimes she would cock her head and wink. Perhaps it was those memories that made her quietly surrender to her fate. The world outside was silent, still and spacious, the kind of space she needed for those last days, for those last heart-warming memories. She had no need for anything more.

Each day that I saw Marie, I asked if she wanted me to take her outside for a little stroll, but she always said, "Oh not today, dear, maybe some other day." But one especially warm autumn day, she asked me. I wrapped a hand-made wool shawl around her and placed the afghan from her bed on her lap, for she was always cold, even in the summer. She asked me to put lipstick on her and comb her hair.

Outside, we sat by a water fountain, listening to the quiet trickling sound of water, watching sunlight sparkle on olive trees. From time to time a warm breeze blew over us. Its gentle motion swayed the slender white-green leaves, leaving long, flickering shadows on the pavement. The fruit had already ripened and fallen. Black stains covered the cement. "The trees are beautiful, aren't they?" Marie said while gazing up at its branches and beyond to the sky. "There is not one cloud today. It's so perfectly clear and blue."

Then she became quiet for a long time. I did not want to disturb her reverie, so I let her sit with the silence until she turned to me and said, "You know, I was in China once, and it was one of the happiest times in my life. Joe was with me. It was our last trip together."

She described the landscape with rice paddies and how the people rose at dawn to do *tai chi* in the fields. "They live a long life there," she said before falling into another silence that was broken by, "Yes, it was one of the happiest times of my life." Then she asked me to take her back inside. She was finished and ready to go back.

This was the first time I had heard about her travels in China. It was the only story she never repeated, as if she were saving it for last. That week she began to decline rapidly, and by the end of the week she had passed away. I wondered if she remembered that happiest time in her life in China when she took her last breath, or did she see Joe at the edge of her bed with his arms wide open, ready to take her on another journey?

Further thoughts

Many elders have to keep busy all the time. It gives them a purpose to go on living. I work with one elder who at 89 still drives, creates art, designs jewelry, goes on travel expeditions around the world, gets a weekly massage and acupuncture treatment, does tai chi every morning, and plays the cello. I admire her spirit and her vitality, and hope I'm able to do the same. I also admire and respect the choices of those who enter their elder years wanting to do less and to create more time for silence and introspection.

Avoid imposing your will, even though your intentions may be good.

Learn to recognize when it might be helpful to encourage your elder to be more social and involved, and when it might not be. Sometimes it is hard to tell the difference between someone who is depressed and self-isolating due to life transitions and someone who simply wants to be left alone with more time for introspection. Consult with all family members, though conflicts sometimes arise as to what is best for mom or dad. This is where working with a team of professionals can be helpful.

CHAPTER
25

AGING IN AMERICA

Essential points

♦ Be a pro-ager.
♦ Be an advocate for aging with grace, dignity, and wisdom.
♦ Learn to bring honor and respect to our elders.
♦ Learn to cultivate and see beauty in the eternal light within.

Why does our society not honor its elders? They do not have a place here as is in other cultures. When you grow old, you become useless and a burden is the message I get from our culture. Just recently I voted and noticed that many ballot measures were for the benefit of children and youth, but not one measure would benefit our elders. Do we really not value them?

While youth is praised and glorified, old age, death, and things associated with death and sickness are neatly kept out of view as if it's better to not see them because they remind us too much of our own mortality. Even a national senior organization continues to promote the message. Nearly every cover model on their monthly magazine has had a face lift and other surgical alterations that fight the aging process rather than embrace it.

Anti-aging is the new lingo, except there is nothing new about it. It has always been in place, except it is wrapped in a slightly different way. If you have money you can grow young again.

We need a new model to embrace. Pro-aging.

I once worked in a community where after loading up a bus of skilled nursing elders for an afternoon drive, I folded the wheel chairs and set them off neatly to the side in the capacious lobby. When my supervisor saw this, she darted toward me brandishing her fists and reprimanding me for putting the wheelchairs there. I apologized, explaining that I thought they were out of the way. She replied, "It's not that! It looks like a bunch of sick old people live here, like some kind of an old age home."

"Oh, really?" I said, bewildered. Not long afterwards I gave my two week notice.

Many cultures do honor their elders and seek them out for their wisdom, such as the Native Americans, the Tibetans and other Asian cultures. In India, growing old and death are simply part of the cycle of life. There is no denial or pretending. By the river, a place that is sacred for many Indians, people pray, worship, bathe, go there to die and to be cremated; and at the same time, children laugh and play, teenage boys and girls fly kites and play games.

An Indian friend told me about a neighboring family where several generations lived together in the same house. The great grandmother, affectionately called Naniji, had become *senile*. She sat in the same room every day, in the same chair, rocking back and forth by the open window next to a towering mango tree, where all day she laughed her wild laugh between mumbling, incoherent phrases. Each family member touched her feet as they had always done to show respect because she was the elder. Life simply went on, just as it was.

When my husband and I traveled to Ladakh, a Tibetan community in India, I could not help but admire the beauty of those old, venerable ones who live long, strong, healthy lives and continue to be a vital part of the community. They may not have had teeth, their faces may have been weathered and wrinkled, yet there was an incredible beauty that came from their eyes. Their remarkable history was written within those wrinkles, telling the story of a resilient, compassionate, peace-loving people living at one with all things and moving with the ebb and flow of the seasons, without fighting, without resistance.

During the winter, the icy season of blizzards when temperatures can drop as low as 20 degrees Centigrade, they are prepared to endure whatever hardships may follow, whatever lessons may be gleaned. There is complete acceptance of what is, of what simply is...

Suggestions for creating engaging and inspiring activities

Facilitate a group of elders who share their experiences of growing older.

Some questions to consider asking:

- Where are you right now in your life? In the grand scheme of things?
- How do you understand your life?
- What is important to you right now?
- What has your life been about?
- What do you want to leave behind?
- How do you want to be remembered?
- What are your fears?

Some questions to ask yourself as a professional or family caregiver:

- How do I feel about my own aging? About becoming ill and needing assistance? About death?
- How do I feel about those closest to me growing old? Dying?

- How do these feelings influence the way I relate to my elders?

CHAPTER 26

FEEDING TUBES AND END OF LIFE

Essential points

◆ Discuss any last wishes and end of life decisions with your loved ones.
◆ Reflect on your own wishes, and let them be known.

> *And in the end, it's not the years in your life that count. It's the life in your years.*

–author unknown, falsely attributed to
Abraham Lincoln

After I opened the double doors, I saw the artificial light, heard the buzzing of florescent light, and smelled the fetid odor of wet diapers that one nurse once described as *wilting stargazer flowers*. They are one of my favorite flowers, yet I cannot help but think that there may be some truth in her description. After taking a few short steps, I came to the nurse's station, and then to a room with three beds. In one bed was Marion, a 99-year-old woman, on her back, not turned nearly enough, not cared for nearly enough and on feeding tubes.

Marion was the first person I saw each day. Sometimes her eyes were open and staring vacantly into the distance, but most of the time they were closed. In the two years that I worked at this community, I never saw her get up from that bed. She could not walk. When her weekly bathing day came, she was probably lifted up onto the Hoyer lift and taken to the shower room. I imagine that was the only time she got up. I don't even think she was ever taken to the beauty parlor. Nearly all her waking and sleeping hours were spent in that bed with rails on both sides, in her powder blue nursing gown, with her sparse white hair hanging to her shoulders.

Sometimes I would rest my hand ever so gently on her hand, knowing how frail her skin was and how it could easily tear and bruise. Her sparse flesh hung like loose chicken skin around the bones of her arms, which were covered with blood clots and bruised-up scabs. Each time I touched her, I shivered because I felt how tender and fragile those arms were. I felt their pain and discomfort. She never spoke. She lived day in and day out in that bed, with the painful, burning sensation of bed sores.

Two good friends, I was told used to visit her once a week, but those visits dwindled to once every two months. It was awkward for the friends, who didn't know what to do or say anymore. They would hold her hand and caress her forehead and hair. Maybe that was the one and only thing that she needed or cared to have. Maybe that was one of her last pleasures.

I heard her friends on more than one occasion say, shaking their heads in dismay, "What a shame. She would not have wanted this. Doesn't her son know? I remember her even saying once how she would never want to be hooked up to a machine."

Marian's eyes suddenly flashed open. Without moving her head, her eyes turned in their direction. Her parched gray-blue lips parted slightly as if she wanted to say something, but she could not speak. Her face was expressionless, yet her eyes implored. She understood, but perhaps her friends did not know that hearing is the last sense to go.

The friends knew more than Marian's son may have known. He was the one who had made the decision to keep her on feeding tubes.

It was a hard decision, especially because he was alone and all decisions rested on his shoulders. On the one hand, you feel it is your duty to preserve life. Life is sacred, and your mother has brought you into this world, has *given you life.*

It can be hard to let go of your mother or any loved one. There is a great attachment and a deep sadness in having to let go. After much deliberation, her son made the decision he felt was best: preserve her life with plugs and a machine.

Every so often, the clear plastic tubes fill with a yellowish, brown liquid that provides Marion with nutrition that she spits up from time to time. Unless a caregiver or someone notices, she can lie there for over an hour in bed in her own expelled matter. I could not help wondering if her son knew what her friends knew, yet still could not bear to let her go.

PART IX

THE BITTERSWEET TRANSIENCE OF LIFE

CHAPTER

27

WE'RE ALL JUST
VISITORS PASSING THROUGH

Essential Points

♦ Create a sacred space for your elders.
♦ Create a space that brings comfort.
♦ Learn to surrender to the process of life, and ultimately death.

> *A famous rabbi in Europe, known for his vast learning and wisdom, was sought out by people from all over the world. One day a man traveled from New York to see him. Expecting the rabbi to live in a lavish dwelling, he was surprised when he saw that the rabbi lived in an attic, with only a bed, a chair, and a few books.*
>
> *"Rabbi, where are your things?" he asked.*
>
> *The rabbi asked in return, "Where are yours?"*
>
> *"I'm only passing through," his visitor replied.*
>
> *The master answered, "So am I, so am I."*

(story adapted from *A Path with Heart*, Jack Kornfield, p.15-16)

I always think of Helena on cold, windy days when my husband and I go for a hike because it is then that I wear a hand-made beige hat, crocheted with nodules that remind me of little marbles or bubbles on bubble wrap. They have a whimsical, playful quality. A tassel tops the hat, and hidden at the back where it gets folded over is a little hole that keeps expanding each time I wear it. It is not a hat that I would normally wear, much less choose for myself, but it is a hat that has become dear to me, a hat that holds a deeper meaning, because it is connected with Helena.

She once loved to knit and crochet and could spend hours making things: blankets, scarves, socks, slippers, shawls, and hats. Her largest drawer was filled with them, yet that was just a fraction of what she had made. The rest she had given away.

One day, she wheeled herself over to her bureau, bending over with a wheezing drawl to open the bottom drawer. Although she spent the next few minutes trying to catch her breath, she didn't seem to mind because she was proud of her work, as she rummaged through an assortment of scarves and blankets. "Look," she said, "here are some of the things I've made." My hands dipped into the soft, warm fluff of yarn, mixed with unexpected bristly textures that smelled of mothballs and old newspapers.

"You were one busy lady, Helena!" I exclaimed.

"I did a lot in my day," she replied, still trying to catch her breath. Most of her items were standard and fairly traditional, just like my mother used to make, many in winter colors like beige, brown, navy blue, and black, but a couple of blankets were bright and vibrant, pulsing with exotic life, emerald green with jagged, zig zag, flaming orange shapes that resembled unfinished lizards or alligators. She loved South America and had lived there for a short while with her husband. Her love came out in the blanket.

"Wow!" I said, touching its surface, which wasn't quite as soft as the other pieces. It had a more bristly, harder, feel. Then I picked up another and another. "These are beautiful." I said.

"Oh, do you really like them?" she asked.

"Yes, of course I do," I replied.

"Then I will give you one. Which one would you like?"

I thought about it. I had plenty of scarves at home, and although the colorful and lively blanket was beautiful, I had more than my fair share of blankets. My mother covered that department, and I had so many that I didn't know where to put them all. Many were stored in plastic bags under the bed. But I did not have a hat, and I remembered how often I wished I had one while hiking on those cold, windy days.

I chose a hat that reminded me of Helena, of something that she would have worn; even the color she often wore. When I saw the hole, I knew it would keep expanding because its threads had grown thin and worn. This hat had lived a full life, yet that made it more special. It held Helena's life, one I would never know as she knew.

The hat also reminded me that nothing lasts forever. All things fade, come to an end and pass. All things transform into something else, take on another shape and form, like the caterpillar turning into the butterfly, or cow dung that fertilizes the soil to help produce a rich harvest of crops, or the seedling that is planted to become a tree or flower.

Within each thread of that hat, Helena's stories were held, even within the worn-out threads that have dissolved into the hole — her stories about the little watch repair store that she and her husband had for many years in New York, as well as stories about their final move to California, where they spent the last few years of their life until his passing a few months earlier.

Helena missed Sam deeply. They had been inseparable from their high school days. He was her one and only love. Shortly after he passed away, her health began to decline, and she needed more care, so she moved from their apartment in independent living into skilled nursing.

Although she had turned her room into a cozy place, having brought many of her own possessions, like the bureau, a velveteen easy chair, an old beige lampshade still speckled with dust, and pictures that filled every inch of space — pictures of her son and daughter, but most were of Helena and Sam from the time of their wedding up until the most recent years — I always got the sense that she knew this was temporary. She was not planning on staying very long. Her time was limited. She took only the most essential things, like the photos. And the rest, she left behind because she knew she was just passing through. How long would she be there? She did not know, but each day, she knew, could be the last, yet I never got the sense that she was holding on for dear life. She accepted her destiny — the destiny, really, of us all.

A short time it was: six months.

Most of her time was spent in bed sleeping or reading. By her bed she kept a stack of books that I got from the library. When she wasn't immersed in a novel, she loved to talk. I sat on the edge of her bed, listening to her stories. She didn't like attending most activities, but she loved anything that had to do with travel, history, art, literature, or poetry.

She loved museums, so I organized some outings with her in mind. I would remind her the day before, and again in the morning. It wasn't that she would forget, but it was a task that required great mental and physical preparation. Often she was able to manage, but as the months passed, she was not up for doing much of anything at all. The art director tried getting her more involved in painting. She sustained an interest for a while, but even that became cumbersome for her. She was more tired and her breathing had become even more labored. She had a hard time using her walker, even for short periods, and had to be in a wheelchair.

In the last weeks, she did not want to leave her bed at all. My room visits began to lessen. She wanted to sleep more, and I sensed that when she wasn't sleeping, she had no more words to speak. Words required too much effort, and she had said all that needed to be said.

She knew that she would be leaving all this behind, and it too required preparation: the preparation that begins with detachment. She began to have less need for outer things to keep her busy. She even lost interest in eating, an activity she had once thoroughly enjoyed. Her trays were often pushed aside and left untouched. She no longer read. It was simply enough to sleep, with memories of her husband surrounding her.

She had once taken pleasure in looking at those nicely framed, old black and white wedding photos and proudly showing them to visitors, with each one opening up another marvelous story. Yet in those last days as she struggled for breath, the photos and stories no longer even mattered. It was as if the prints held within frame and glass had faded from her sight. Maybe the spirit held within them was what was left imprinted on her heart. That she could take with her. Then again, maybe that will fade too. I do not know, really.

I do know that whenever I wear that old, worn hat on cold, windy days while hiking with my husband up narrow, steep, damp paths through forests of eucalyptus and pine, I remember Helena and her life as it passed quickly before me, and I remember that we are all just visitors passing through. The thought does not frighten me. It makes me embrace life even more and love each day for whatever it brings. What I am more afraid of is not having lived my life as fully as I would have liked and not having pursued my dreams.

Further thoughts

Creating the right space is important for both those preparing to die and for those still vibrant and thriving. Our space reflects who we are, where we are, and what we want in life. If we want our elders to be inspired and creative, we should help set up a space that makes them feel inspired and creative. And if like Helena, our elder is preparing for death, we should help create a space that brings comfort.

Encourage your loved one to make her creative space special, a place of retreat and comfort, a sacred space where he can connect to his deepest self — whatever that may mean to him or her. Every individual is different. For example, before I write, give a massage, or do anything creative, I like to take a few moments to meditate, or to say a little prayer that the divine will work through me. I have an altar with photos of people who have inspired me. I like to light candles and incense. For me that is what makes my space sacred, and I set my intention. For someone else it may mean setting a positive intention; playing a certain piece of music; dedicating his space or project to someone dear; placing a photo of someone who inspires her; or a putting a fresh flower in a vase. These are all ways of honoring the creative process.

NOW IS THE TIME
AND NOT A MOMENT LATER

Essential points

♦ Trust your intuitive voice.
♦ Celebrate accomplishments.
♦ Honor wisdom.
♦ See the beauty and goodness in all things.

> *And if not now, when?*
>
> Rabbi Hillel
> *Pirkei Avot 1:14*

Each time I stepped into her room I heard a small voice say, *Do it now, don't put it off until later.* The first time was in the beginning of October, then every time thereafter, from the first glimpse outside the hallway to the first step over her threshold.

Entering her room was like entering another world filled with magic, color, vibrancy, and pulsing with a love for life. Sheila was an artist in her spare time, when she was not busy raising three children and taking care of the house.

Years ago she had stopped painting, but her paintings were everywhere. Every inch of space on her wall was covered. Her style reminded me of Grandma Moses' naïve, yet refreshing simplicity, yet when you looked closely at each painting, you began to see its complexity. Individual blades of grass spread out on a canvas of open countryside, with perfectly round rolling hills, and dandelion-shaped trees, little black v-shaped birds nestled within the leafy puff of branches set against azure skies, flocks of birds flying into white clouds shaped like happy flowers — big, bright, and bouncy — and cheerful, glowing suns.

It was hard to feel sad while looking at Sheila's paintings. Daffodils, daisies and sunflowers spread out like happy faces laughing in the sun, while shouting the message, *Hey, look at me! I am here to make you smile. This is my purpose.* There were also serene, idyllic seascapes with sandcastles and children's plastic pails filled with seashells and pearls, and birds with exotic plumes perched within rows of coconut palms.

"These are gorgeous!" I gushed.

Each time I said those words during that particular October, I kept hearing the little voice say, *Do it now, do a special exhibit of her work, do not delay, ask her now, not later.* Under normal circumstances I would have heeded the voice, but it was an overwhelmingly busy time. I was working closely with an elder who was put on hospice, as well as on another resident's art show. I was planning an important journey to India, and was scheduled to leave in a little over three weeks. In preparation for the trip, I had been taking extra time off work.

But something in me told me each time I saw her to *Do it now*, and to not delay, yet there was another voice that kept saying *Not now, I'm too busy! Better to wait until I get back. Besides, she never is interested in participating in activities.* Indeed, whenever

I saw a program that I thought Sheila would enjoy, I asked her and she always declined by saying, "Oh honey, not today…"

But the voice kept persisting, *NOW, DO IT NOW, NOT LATER,* while the other voice battled, *Why now, what's the hurry?* After all, Sheila did look healthy and well. In fact, she looked beautiful. Although she rarely came out of her room in the two years I had been there, she never looked unwell.

She liked to say, "It's old age, dear. I'm weary. Just getting up and out of bed to sit in a wheelchair is a strain for me." Yet she really was beautiful for a 99-year-old woman. Still round and curvaceous, she had barely a wrinkle on her clear skin. There was a little sagging around the eyes and jaw, but her flawlessly radiant face was topped with a full head of silver gray hair that was always nicely fixed with curls. Somehow, she managed to muster the strength to go to the in-house beauty parlor once a week to have her hair and nails done.

"These bones are old and tired," she would say through a sigh. Other than that, she was lively and loved to talk. She was curious about people, and whenever I came to visit her, she asked a lot of questions.

"What are you doing these days, darling? Are they keeping you busy here? How is your husband? Is he well? He sounds like such a wonderful man."

"He is a wonderful man, and he *is* doing well!" I replied. I would tell her a story, and the following week or month she would remember the story with all its details. She even knew of my love for India and how I had been planning this trip for a long time.

Each time I talked with her during that particular October, she said, "You must be excited about your trip, honey; it's getting closer, isn't it?"

"Closer than I like to think. It's a big journey, and time is racing."

"How many more days now, is it?" she asked.

"Twenty-two, from this day." I replied.

"Well you'll have to tell me all about it, once you come back." I could hear the battle beginning again, with one voice saying, *Do it now, don't delay* and the other voice saying, *Now is not the right time. You're too busy! You know how much planning and preparation an art show takes.*

One day the little voice won. On impulse, while talking to Sheila about India, I blurted, "I'd love to do a special art exhibit of all your paintings with a reception. What do you think? Are you up for it?"

A part of me was hoping that she would decline, but this time, without thought or question, she replied, "I would love to. I'm honored."

For the next three weeks, I prepared for two very important days: the day of my departure to India on Nov. 2, and Sheila's art show on October 31.

Sheila counted the days. Whenever I saw her, the big question was no longer, "How many more days until you leave for India?" but "How many more days until the show?"

It went from two weeks to 10 days to seven to four, until the day came when I declared, "Tomorrow is the big day."

"Well, I'm just delighted," she replied. "I'm all ready, you know. All I have to do is gather the strength to get up, have my hair done, and be there."

I knew how difficult it was for her. What may take me five minutes to do could take Shelia three hours. When the following day came she woke up bright and early instead of sleeping to her usual 10 or 11 o'clock. She informed her caregiver that she not only wanted to go to the beauty parlor, but also wanted to be dressed up in her finest and made up to look more beautiful than ever.

When the time of her show came, I thought I would have to come to her room and get her, but she wheeled herself. I was stunned! That required a lot of strength and energy, but she had the will and intention to fulfill her important mission.

The drab, dark dining room had been transformed. Tables were pushed together to make one long table covered with gold satin cloth, where I displayed all her paintings. Fresh flowers, silver platters with hors d'oeuvres, and plastic flutes for champagne and apple cider were set out on other tables draped with cloth.

I had invited staff, residents from skilled nursing and independent living, all her family members, and the art teacher with whom she had developed a close friendship. Unfortunately, as much as her family would have liked to have been there because they adored and loved her, they were not able to come because they were spread out across the country, with one living in Europe. I knew that although Sheila would have liked them to have been there, she understood how hard it was for them, and she would make this a special day anyway. It was *her day*.

I was so proud of her when I saw the grace and confidence with which she carried herself. Wheeling herself down the aisle among the clamor of wheelchairs, she glowed. She looked around, as if taking everything and everyone in as fully as possible. She was not used to seeing the dining room this elegant, nor filled with this kind of festive spirit.

Sheila was pleased with how her paintings were displayed. And how delightfully surprised she was when she saw all the people who came to honor her! The room was packed with all her friends, staff, acquaintances, and residents.

Applause, loud claps, soft ones, hurrahs, and whistles resounded, bringing renewed life to that room in that hour. Moved, Sheila took it all in, beaming, ready to show the world what she was about, what she had done with her hands, some paints, and a brush on canvass. I was so touched, tears came to my eyes. I also saw tears in the eyes of other elders.

My plan was to ask Sheila a whole set of questions. Instead, she elaborated with such eloquence on the first one, "What inspires you?" that new questions were spawned, one leading to the next, with a room filled with hands rising, hands shaking in *Pick me, pick me, I have a question*.

"Where were you born?"

"Louisiana."

"Did you go to college to study art?"

"No, I went for two years to college to study accounting, but never finished. I met my husband, and that was that!" she said playfully, a twinkle in her eyes, as if reflecting on that life-changing moment. There was not a bit of regret.

She spoke about the importance of her family, and how they were her inspiration, especially her grandchildren, who were now all grown. "Not a day passed," she said, "when I did not learn something from the children. I saw how they looked at the world with such wonder. Everything around them, from the grass to the trees, to the flowers and birds and bugs, to the sea and the waves in the sea, made them curious. In painting, the same kind of curiosity and wonder is required. With every subject, I've learned to look as if through their eyes, and as if for the first time, although I may have studied the subject over a hundred times."

I will never forget her words. She talked about the importance of seeing beauty and goodness in all things. Maybe that was why she had lived to be 99 and still looked so beautiful. Maybe that was why those paintings made everyone feel so happy. I could well imagine that even if those landscapes had in reality been dismal, dark and unhappy, she would have infused them with beauty and life because that was how she saw the world. I am sure those paintings always reminded her of the goodness and beauty in *all* things, even within the setting of skilled nursing and in spite of a fragile and ailing body. She was shining her light to all people who were present on that day.

After the show, she lingered to talk with friends over a small glass of red wine. When she was finished, I could see that the energy required for the day had completely dissipated. She was ready to retire. I helped her back to her room, and she and was in bed by 5:30.

"I'm so happy that we were able to do this, Sheila," I said, while pausing from putting her paintings back on the walls.

She was not yet sleeping, just resting, as if still taking in the magnificence of the day. With a depth and seriousness in her eyes, like I had never seen before, she replied in a tone both heartfelt and weary, "So am I, dear. So am I." I stood frozen, my eyes connecting with hers. For one split second, she moved her head. A glare came from her glasses. Her eyes were momentarily hidden from view, but when she tilted her head again, ever so slightly, I saw the light in her eyes again, bright yet fading. I could not find the words to reply. I was breathless. The moment was filled with a depth, both electrifying and intense. It was haunting. "So am I, dear. So am I."

After a long sigh, I said, "I'm glad, I'm so glad. Thank you for sharing your work and life today. Thank you."

"It was my pleasure. You have quite an important day ahead of you too! You'll be leaving for India soon!"

"Yes, in two days."

"You'll have to tell me all about it when you come back dear."

"Yes, Sheila, I will," I said, hanging the last painting on her wall before saying my last goodnight. Two weeks later, while I was in India, Sheila passed away.

Further thoughts

What a difference it makes to feel seen, heard, and valued for the wisdom one has gathered through many years of living. How empowering!

Suggestions for creating engaging and inspiring activities

♦ Organize a wisdom circle where the elders share their life lessons. You might consider using a talking stick, a Native American custom. When each one is finished speaking, he or she ends with, "And I have spoken…" and passes the stick to the next elder. A favorite object can be used in place of a stick.

♦ When the weather is warm, go to the park or other natural setting where the elders can ponder the life lessons they would like to leave to the next generation. Since many elders may not be able to write, I suggest keeping a notebook or recorder to record what they share. Every week you'll gather more wisdom teachings until you'll have enough to create a little book of treasured wisdom.

♦ Make this book of wisdom a celebratory event. Invite family members, community staff, and larger community and ask the elders to share their wisdom. Make it intergenerational by inviting your local high school.

♦ Dedicate the book to those who have been instrumental in shaping the elders' wisdom. Gratitude is so important.

♦ Organize a fund raiser. Keep the book on display at your community.

Some questions to consider asking your elders:

♦ What were some major losses or difficulties in your life that made you stronger and wiser?

♦ What did you learn from each experience?

♦ Who or what were some of the teachers in your life? Review your life from childhood through your elder years. Remember that teachers can be anyone or anything that we learn from: our pets, our children, strangers, neighbors, a beggar in the street, an event, or any experience that left a major imprint.

♦ What advice would you give about love, home keeping, money, and career?

♦ What are your highest values? Have they changed over time? If so, how have they changed?

♦ What advice would you give to a young person struggling with identity, self-esteem, or confusion over what he or she may want to do in life?

29

THE LAST DAYS WITH ROSIE

Essential Points

- Be a source of comfort.
- Bring presence; listen wholeheartedly.
- Learn to love, give, grieve, yet be able to let go.
- Resolve to clear up any unfinished business with your loved ones.

"Cooookie, Cooookie," Rosie yelled from her room in a sing-song tone, with the *coooo* crescendoing to a higher pitch that diminished with a drawl on the *kie*. Funny, the only time Rosie called out the name "cookie" was when she sensed I was near. Her room could be completely quiet, but the minute I turned the corner near her room or stepped quietly into my office across the hall, her endearing calls of *coooookie* began.

Rosie knew that I had a soft spot for her and that whenever she yelled *coookie*, I would come running when everyone else was too busy. Often I dropped everything to rush to her aid, although at times she had the same request over and over again, like needing assistance to the toilet, even though her caregiver had just helped her. I would remind her that she just went.

"Are you sure, Cookie?" she would ask.

"I'm sure," I replied.

Cookie was what she called me because she always forgot my real name. I didn't mind. I kind of liked being called Cookie. She was the kind of person who everyone adored and wanted to help. But sweet and cute as she was, she was a feisty little thing with a lot of spunk. Every day she asked me to find her a newspaper. She especially liked the *Wall Street Journal,* but any newspaper would do, so long as the business section was included Finances, the stock market, NASDAQ, those were the kinds of things she was interested in. The rest she would leave.

Hastily thumbing through the pages, she would pull out the business section and sit back in her propped-up bed, wearing glasses that looked like goggles on her puckered-up, face. She knew what she wanted in the world and how to get it. Always did, and always would. Her approach worked, especially with me.

At times Rosie was like a good friend, at other times like a sister. One day, with our hands intertwined, she said, "I feel like you're my sister, like we have a long history together. Just think, if I could get out of this bed right now, we could travel to India together." She knew I had just recently returned from India, and she loved to travel.

After her husband passed away, Rosie traveled around the world with her only sister, of whom she was fond. But India was one place she had never been. She wanted to know all about the trip, what the people were like, where I stayed, and what drew me there. I told her that I was writing a book and doing research.

"Oh, I see," she said, "and what got you interested in India?" I told her I had studied Indian philosophy and religion.

"What an interesting subject. If I were to write a book, that's what I would choose to write about. Religion and God."

"What would you say?" I asked.

"That people make too much fuss over what they are, the religion they are, and not enough about who they are. Are they good? Are they kind? Do they bring good to the world? Those are the important things. I believe in a god, but I also believe that God does not claim him or herself as the one and only god for a particular group of people. One says, I'm right, the other says, no I'm right, you're wrong. Maybe they are all right and we should be quiet and not make such a fuss over it. I bet you have a similar view. Is that what your book is about?"

"Well, it's not really a book about religion. It's a novel."

"Oh? About what?" she asked.

"It's about a young woman who keeps having dreams of a holy place in India, where two rivers meet to become one after miles of separation. Inspired by the visions, she begins writing a story set there. After a year, she suddenly stops without understanding why and is unable to finish the story, when unexpectedly an invitation comes. She is invited to India, along with four friends. At the time of the invitation, she does not know that it is the same place as her unfinished story. A series of unexpected events unfold, including the sudden death and cremation of one of the friends, which leads to a spiritual awakening, as well as the completion of the unfinished story."

"Are you the woman?"

"Well, in part, but not entirely. There are always some elements of truth woven with fiction."

"But how did you get so interested in India?"

"When I was a little girl, my father showed me pictures of this strange yet alluring land. I was fascinated by the images I saw — magnificent statues of the Buddha, and cows wandering side by side with the people and cars in the streets, and temples with dancing gods, animal gods, and gods with many faces. That year my father died and I was too young to really understand death, yet I understood the sadness that separation brings. As a way of dealing with the inexplicable sadness I suddenly felt, I escaped in my imagination to this place in the pictures. I knew that I had to go there someday, yet I did not know at that time that the land was called India."

"Is that in your book?"

"It's a part of the story, yes."

"How old were you when he died?"

"Four."

"What a shame," she said, shaking her head back and forth. "Just like my son. His father died when he was seven. I had to raise him all on my own."

"In spite of it, you did a wonderful job! And so did my mother!"

"Did she work?"

"She was a church organist, but then she had to find another job in a candy factory. What about you?"

"After my husband died, I worked as a bookkeeper."

"You and my mother are heroes — remember that, Rosie. True heroes. Look at your son. He's a wonderful man." And he was. He came every day to visit her with some special little treat, like a Starbuck's coffee, a milkshake, or a box of candy, among an assortment of other goodies that she sometimes requested. He was always so appreciative of the time I spent with his mother.

"And you know, I never remarried. I did it all my own," she said, nodding her head, proudly.

I knew how much Rosie loved her son. He was the most important thing in her life, especially after her husband passed away. More than anyone else, Rosie reminded me deeply of my mother, who also chose not to remarry. I wondered if that choice was a part of the way that generation thought. Rosie, like my mother, also got married and gave birth later in life when she was in her mid-40s, and that certainly was not common for women of that generation.

I remember the first time I met her, the day she arrived from the hospital on a stretcher, still recovering from surgery after having fallen and broken her hip. Although she was heavily sedated, she was in a lot of pain, as well as incoherent and disoriented. Immediately transferred to a bed with steel guard-rails to prevent her from falling, she spent the next three months in that room, her new home. It was late afternoon in January.

Repeatedly she called, "Mama, Mama, Mama." Her voice held an incredible amount of pain, loneliness, and longing that always brought tears to my eyes. Something about the tone of her voice reminded me of my love for my own mother and the longing that I sometimes feel for her. There was something about her too that reminded me of my mother, but I couldn't explain why, because they did not look alike; yet it connected us deeply from the very first day. Each time I heard her call "Mama," I could not help but run to her side to see what I could do for her. I was prepared to do whatever possible to ease her suffering.

She moved her head back and forth on the pillow repeating, "Mama, Mama, help me, help me." I noticed how incredibly thin she was. Her chest was sunken, her ribs protruding. She broke my heart.

"I'm here to help you," I whispered, while touching her frail hand with its thin, loose flesh severely bruised, as were the rest of her arms.

"Mama, Mama, Mama," she cried again, her voice strained and tired.

"My name is Mary Ann, and I'm here to help you. Tell me what you need," I replied in a soft voice, gently pressing my other hand to her forehead.

"I'm in pain," she said, with her hands near her lower abdomen. "Right here, I'm in pain."

"I'll get a nurse," I said and went to tell the nurse, who said Rosie was just given pain medication. I let Rosie know that that her pain should subside in few moments.

"I'm hungry, Mama." Her tray was left untouched. She did not have teeth or dentures, and I wondered how she would ever eat the hamburger sitting in front of her.

"I will bring you some soup," I replied. Promptly I marched to the kitchen and brought her some soup and yogurt, but she pushed it away.

"The pain, Mama, Mama, Mama," she kept saying, but her eyes began to close. The medication must have been kicking in, for her *Mamas* became less and less. I stood by her until I knew she had fallen asleep. That marked the beginning of our heartfelt relationship.

It did not take Rosie long to bounce back to her old self, or at least the lucid self that could converse and express her needs more fully. After a week or so, she surprised me when I came to work on a Monday and saw her sitting in a wheelchair, fully dressed with a pretty white blouse tucked neatly into a pair of black slacks. Her short grey hair was combed back neatly and parted to the side, with her hands folded sweetly in her lap. With childlike wonder, she looked around at the new environment. I could see she was no longer in pain or confusion. She exuded a certain kindness that again reminded me of my mother.

I introduced myself to her again, not knowing whether she would remember me. I asked her about herself. She told me she was born in Russia, but came here when she was a little girl. She lived in Sacramento and had a lovely house where she wanted to return. She was worried that no one would look after her garden. She came here because her son lived in this area.

I introduced her to her neighbors. She was well received immediately. Soon she was busy chatting with her new friends, but Rosie never saw herself as fitting in with the others. One day with her hand covering her mouth, she whispered, "Look at all these old people! I'm surrounded by them. What am I doing here? I don't belong." Delighted, I could not help but smile at this 99-year-old, adorable woman sitting before me.

Taking her face in between my hands, I said, "I love you Rosie. You are wonderful. And no, you don't belong here, but I'm glad you're here anyway so that I could get to know you better."

In so many ways, Rosie kept reminding me of my mother, who would have said something similar. In the last days of my mother's life, I went to the hospital to take her home and brought her a change of clothes and a pair of shoes.

"Where did you pick these up?" my 80-year-old mother exclaimed, looking at the shoes aghast. "They look like old lady shoes."

"They were in your closet, Mama."

"Well, gee whiz. I don't know how they got there. I would never wear shoes like that." I wondered if her reaction had something to do with her young and handsome male nurse.

One day, my mother looked so angelic while resting peacefully in her hospital bed when suddenly she opened her eyes and frantically cried out, "What time is it?"

"Three' o clock, Mom."

"Where are my dentures? Get me my comb. Jim will be here any minute."

"Jim?" I asked. "Who's Jim?"

Before this, I never saw my mother flirt, much less go out with a man. That was something she would never dream of, or so I thought.

"He's the nurse who comes on duty at three to give me my medications." Sure enough, shortly after three, with Mom's dentures in, her short gray hair combed and parted neatly on the side, Mom smiled coquettishly as Jim came in the room. "You must be here to give me my shots, Jim," she said sweetly.

"Yes, I am, Ceil," he said playfully. After some bantering he asked for her arm.

"Anything, Jim," she said, batting her eyes, her arm extended. "Anything you want."

I wondered if I were dreaming. My mother flirtatious? The good Catholic woman who never dreamed of remarrying, who prayed fervently to the Virgin Mary, and whom I had never seen flirt with any man, was flirting with a man, less than half her age, and he was flirting right back with her.

While Rosie was never flirtatious like my mother, she was charming and immediately won the hearts of both male and female nurses. And of course, from the very first moment she won my heart completely. From that day on, I spent time with her. She was the first person I saw in the morning and the last in the evening just before I went home.

Some part of Rosie kept thinking this place was only temporary. One day while resting in bed, she looked up at me and said, "I will miss you. You've become my good friend, but I'll be going home soon. Promise me you'll keep in touch with me. Come see me sometime. Sacramento is not too far, or maybe I'll move in with my son. He lives very close. That will be easier for you."

Thinking there may have been some truth in what she said, I checked with the charge nurse and was informed that when Rosie first came to skilled nursing two months ago, going home was a slight possibility, if her body strengthened enough for her to use a walker, but that never happened. Now, she was being considered for hospice. A wave of sadness hit me. I realized I would have to say goodbye to my dear friend.

Although it was clear she was growing weaker, spending more time in bed and less time getting out of her room, she kept talking about going home and how she would miss me.

"We've only just begun," she said tenderly, "There is still so much for us to learn about each other. I won't be here much longer, but you'll come visit when you have time."

Rosie was right, this place *was* only temporary, yet so was the home in Sacramento where she would never return. Perhaps the home she was speaking of was another one, the one that belongs to us all.

One day I asked her if she was afraid of death.

"No," she replied frankly. "There comes a point in one's life when you become tired, simply tired, and you welcome it. What about you? You see people dying all the time."

"I'm not afraid, but it's always comes as a shock that so and so was here just yesterday and now they are gone. Each time it happens, there is the same jolt, the same sudden awakening that our lives truly pass so quickly. We never know when it will happen, but one thing is for sure: it happens to us all. There is always a part of me that wonders where they are. Can they still hear and see? Is some part of their consciousness still lingering? I think so. What do you think Rosie?"

"I think so too. I don't see death as an end..."

Rosie stopped for a moment, as if thinking about what she would say when her contemplative expression changed suddenly to a buoyant one, eyes twinkling, with that infectious, toothless smile of hers that was terribly sweet and endearing. "Oh, Rosie!" I exclaimed.

"You're just like my sister," she said, patting my hand. "We think alike about a lot of things. Don't you think?"

I couldn't help giving her a kiss on the cheek. She was right. We did think a lot alike. She knew me well and often knew my views on issues before I even expressed them. I wondered if it was because she was perceptive, or if it was because she truly saw in me a sister.

Not long after that conversation, I sat with her while she slept. Her eyes were closed, her clasped hands resting on her chest, as if in a deep, peaceful slumber. Just when I was about to slip quietly away, she popped her head up as if wide awake, opened her eyes, and said, "I love you, Cookie." It was the first time I ever heard her say those words. I was so moved that I almost forgot what to say and how to say it. The words eventually came, though they were choked inside, "I love you too, Rosie."

Her words reminded me of my mother shortly before she died. Just as I was about to walk out the door, my arms filled with laundry, my mother — who appeared to be asleep with her hands clasped on her chest — opened her eyes and called my name. At first she said nothing, but I could see that she was thinking about what she wanted to say, and how she would say it.

"You do know that I love you very much and that I will miss you, don't you? And you do know that I tried to raise you the best way I could, don't you?" The sorrow in her eyes and the way she spoke — with clarity, yet choked with emotion, pausing in between words, pauses that were filled with a certain heaviness — told me that this same heaviness had been burdening her heart for a long time. Yet she had never told me until then. It made me shiver in the summer heat. Something stirred deeply in my heart that made me want to cry.

I dropped the laundry on a chair and sat next to her, slipping my hand into hers. "Yes, of course I do. Of course I do … if there was anything, Mama, that I ever said or did that hurt you, please forgive me too."

"You do know then, how much I love you. You do understand that, don't you?" she said, taking my face in between her hands.

"Yes, I understand that you love me. Do you forgive me?"

"What is past is past," she replied. "We move forward in time, not back."

All my life I had complained. I held petty little grudges, things that had been unresolved within me, which really had nothing to do with my mother. I was critical. She took all that I ever said to heart, but never mentioned it until then. In that moment I felt like the wounded bird caged within my heart was suddenly released and set free and whole again. Whatever grievances I had ever held onto dissolved and no longer mattered.

Nothing mattered except forgiveness and love. I know she did her best, and she loved me more than anyone I will ever know. Within a pause of shared silence, some bigger force was at work. Whatever needed to be healed was healed. I was free, and so was she. They were her last words, just as "I love you" were Rosie's last words to me.

Rosie once said that she had some difficulties with her son. I wondered if they had a moment together, like the one I had with my mother, where last words are spoken, and what needs to said is said. When I asked her about it, she did not seem to want to talk about it, so I let it go.

After her *I love you*, Rosie declined rapidly. Most of the time she slept. My visits continued twice a day, but our conversations were replaced by silence. I simply sat next to her, being present to something bigger that has no words. It was a true gift.

Earlier in the day when Rosie was livelier and spoke those last words to me, she said something else that struck me as odd because it seemed to come out of nowhere, "Be sure to put me in that book of yours."

I was baffled. "What book?" I asked. *How would she fit into a novel about India?* I wondered. *What was she thinking? Did she forget about the book I described?*

"The book you are writing about all these people in here," she replied matter-of-factly, as if I had forgotten and she was reminding me. At the time, this book was not part of the plan.

I did not have the heart to tell Rosie she was not part of the novel, so instead I simply said, "O.K., Rosie, I will."

Little did I know that she saw something I did not see. Three months later, my old supervisor, whom I adored, was unexpectedly replaced by another, and I decided to leave. I grieved the loss immensely, and one evening over dinner with friends, I shared the grief. I expressed how attached I had grown to so many people there, and how I missed them all. Projects had been started that would never get finished.

When I shared the stories of the elders that evening, inspiration stirred over our dinner table. Our friend Raphael said, "You've got to write a book about this. I am going through all this with my mother. I just moved her into an assisted living community. People like me need to hear these stories. They bring hope."

"I've been telling her for years to write these stories," my husband chimed in.

The timing could not have been better. I had put aside the other project to take a break for a while. The more I thought about writing this book, the more appealing it became. While I was thinking about all the elders I had worked with who had come and gone, I realized they continue to live within my heart. By writing a book, I would honor them and they would continue to live on the page.

Rosie was like a bridge from my past —reminding me of how this work began with the death of my mother — to the future. Rosie saw the future that I did not. Two weeks later when she passed away, I felt a sadness and emptiness each time I walked past her room, with its blank space on the door where her name once was, as I realized I would no longer hear her calls of *Cooookie*. Although I had known her death was coming, it came as a shock. As I stood in her room, I wondered, as I always wonder, *does she see, does she hear, does she know I am here in her room with her bed empty, and her night table with an old newspaper opened to the business section, along with her smudged-up glasses, crumbled-up tissues and a box of See's with empty wrappers and half-eaten candy? I will miss you, Rosie, I will miss you.*

Someone once asked me how I could do the work I do. *Don't you get attached? Isn't it hard?* Yes, I do get attached, but I could not imagine having lived my life without knowing Rosie. It was an honor to have her as my friend. It was a true gift being with her in those last days. Whatever sadness may come, it will pass, as all things do, yet the imprint she left within my heart will never fade. Knowing Rosie was a beautiful experience far outweighing the suffering and sadness that come from loss and separation. Suffering and sadness pass, but love remains.

PART X

PLAY, PRESENCE, LAUGHTER AND JOY

THE ETERNAL BLISS OF LAUGHTER

Essential Points

♦ Bring more laughter into your elders' daily life.
Laughter is healing.
♦ Create community through shared laughter.

> *O what is laughter, Hafiz?*
> *What is this precious love and laughter*
> *Budding in our hearts?*
> *It is the glorious sound*
> *Of a soul waking up!*
>
> Hafiz, *I Heard God Laughing*

Loosening the grip on her leather bag held tightly in her lap, Estelle laughed a loud rippling roar that sent electrifying waves through the room. Everyone turned to see who was laughing that unfamiliar laugh, because Estelle was somber, stoic, taciturn. I don't remember *ever* seeing her smile, yet on that day did she *ever* smile and laugh. It was the first time I saw her body, always so stiff and erect, relax with her two hands letting go of the tight grip she always held on her pocketbook, as a stunned silence filled the room. Heads turned, with eyes honing in on Estelle, who sat in the back at the corner table alone wearing her usual tan suit jacket, her white-collared blouse buttoned tightly to her neck.

No one could really see her because she had a way of making herself inconspicuous and was often turned to the side, so we saw her only in profile – straight white hair cropped short and blunt, with sharply chiseled features, aquiline nose, thin lips fading into snow white skin, with barely a wrinkle. Her profile stood against a copy of a Monet painting hanging on the wall: the softly shaped forms of a haystack at midday in the background in shades of gold and rose; light and cheery in and of itself. The painting was made even brighter and lighter by Estelle's laughter.

The silence slipped away into a wave of gasps, *aahs,* and *ohhs, it's Estelle, can you believe it,* in the midst of giggles, chuckles, and whispers reaching out to meet and commingle with her boisterous laugh. Everyone was gathered together for an hour of humor. Nearly all the women were Jewish, so I thought my collection of Jewish jokes would be perfect, including my most recent find of funny typos and slips in synagogue announcements, which I found in *J magazine.* Others found them so funny that I had to pause after each one because they needed time to catch their breath.

Through all this, Estelle was deadpan quiet. It wasn't until the very end of the hour when she let out her rippling roar, but when she did, did she *ever.* Then, waving me over with her long, thin hands, she asked me to tell her the joke again. Eyes agog, we all watched her let out another howl, followed by another.

Before this, I had read at least a dozen jokes, and I can attest it certainly wasn't this one: *Thursday at 9, there will be a meeting of the Little Mothers' club. All women wishing to become Little Mothers, please see the rabbi in his private study.* That one marked the rambunctious beginning of the hour. Nearly all the elders had a grand old time hooting and hollering. One laughed so hard that her dentures flew clear across the room and that made her howl even louder!

A little prankish smile may have curled on Estelle's lips then, but no laughter.

Nor was it this one: *The Men's Club is warmly invited to the oneg hosted by Hadassah. Refreshments will be served for a nominal feel.* That one really set them roaring, with one woman laughing so hard that she farted!

Everyone looked at each other, as if to say *it wasn't me who did it*, and that made them laugh even louder. Another lady, giggling like a schoolgirl, asked through a playful whisper, "Is that really what they said in the announcement?"

"Yes, it really is what they said. Quite a big typo, huh!" I replied.

"Oh my, oh my," she said sweetly, with her plump, wrinkled hand covering her mouth in a fit of delightful, naughty humor. Mirth danced and whirled in the room, yet still no laugh from Estelle.

And it wasn't *this one* either that came somewhere in the middle of the hour:

Don't let worry kill you. Let your synagogue help. Join us for our oneg after services. Prayer and medication to follow. Remember in prayer the many who are sick of our congregation. The group continued laughing just as loud and raucous as ever, with hands slapping knees, and arms holding sides of rolling bellies, with one elder brazenly confessing, "My pants are all wet, I just wee' wee'd from laughing so hard!"

Through all that fun-loving commotion, Estelle sat deadpan quiet, gripping her bag.

Nor was it this one: *A bean supper will be held Wednesday evening in the community center. Music will follow.* In the spirit of glee, tears rolled down one elder's face, as her friend in the wheel chair next to her was busy readjusting her hearing aid so she wouldn't miss a word, which was getting difficult through the high volume of rejuvenating laughter.

I was thrilled and wanted to shout, *yes, laugh and be merry, laugh your way to well being, good health, and happiness.* I thought maybe all this would rub off on Estelle, but still it didn't. I told two more jokes that failed to move her. *If you enjoy sinning, the choir is looking for you,* followed by *the ladies of Hadassah have cast off clothing of every kind and they may be seen in the basement on Tuesdays.*

Finally I told this one: *Why are Jewish men circumcised? Because Jewish women won't touch anything unless they get 20% off.* This was the one that finally did it, releasing a stream of mirthful tears, making her hold the sides of her ribs, loosening her grip on the purse, as everyone paused in amazement.

"Again!" she shouted, a big bright smile twisting her lips. "One more time."

"Yes, yes, yes," I declared, "I will say it again and again."

How happy I was seeing this transformation. How I rejoiced in that moment, bubbling with laughter, along with everyone else for the last few minutes of that blissful hour. Yes, yes, yes!

Further thoughts

Some benefits of laughter include:

- ◆ Stimulates your organs. "Laughter enhances your intake of oxygen-rich air, stimulates your heart, lungs and muscles, and increases the endorphins that are released by your brain." (See the article, *Stress relief from laughter? It's no joke,* at http://www.mayoclinic.org/healthy-lifestyle/stress-management/in-depth/stress-relief/art-20044456?)

- ◆ Soothes tension, stimulates circulation, and aids muscle relaxation, which help relieve some of the physical symptoms of stress. (Mayo Clinic)

♦ "Improves your immune system. Negative thoughts manifest into chemical reactions that can affect your body by bringing more stress into your system and decreasing your immunity. In contrast, positive thoughts actually release neuropeptides that help fight stress and potentially more-serious illnesses." (Mayo Clinic)

♦ Relieves pain by causing the body to produce its own natural painkillers. (Mayo Clinic)

♦ Makes it easier to cope with difficult situations. (Mayo Clinic)

♦ Improves your mood. Makes you happier. Lessens anxiety and depression. (Mayo Clinic)

Suggestions for creating engaging and inspiring activities

♦ Have an hour of humor once a week with jokes and/or funny movies. Laughter can be contagious and healing, as long as it's not at someone else's expense.

♦ Facilitate a laughter yoga club. Laughter Yoga was created by Dr. Madan Kataria, a medical doctor who was inspired by his findings while researching the benefits of laughter on the human mind and body. The first laughter yoga club started in 1995 with only 5 people in a park in Mumbai, India, and has spread over the last 20 years across India and throughout the world. It has been used in hospitals, prisons and senior care facilities with great success.

♦ Celebrate World Laughter Day every year on the first Sunday in May. In 1998, Dr. Kataria created World Laughter Day to promote world peace. "When you laugh, you change and when you change, the whole world changes around you."

♦ See http://www.laughteryoga.org for more information on Dr. Kataria's work and laughter yoga

For family caregivers

♦ Find a few simple items that make your loved one chuckle: pictures, a comic strip, a joke in print; and hang them on a wall in a visible place.

♦ Keep a collection of funny movies around.

PLAY AND BE PRESENT

Essential Points

When with an individual who has Alzheimer's:

- Encourage her to engage in activities she can enjoy and feel successful doing.
- Praise small accomplishments.
- Don't criticize what she cannot do.
- Learn to play.
- Bring joy.
- Be present.
- Leave your problems at home.

> *What, then, is the right way of living? Life must be lived as play.*
>
> Plato, *Laws*

Play and be present ... these are the words that come to mind when I think of Daisy, but there are other words that come to mind as well, like *whimsical, spontaneous, alive, frolic and romp, fun-loving and free, uninhibited, child-like wonder and awe, delight, effervescent and bubbly, bouncy, imaginative,* and *delicious laughter mixed with bird song on a spring day.*

*Be present and play...*That was how I worked with Daisy, never *thinking too much* about *what* we were doing, but *trusting* in the *present moment*...Daisy had Alzheimer's and had lost the ability to verbalize, except for mumbo jumbo, but her body was expressive, and her face talked all the time. I knew when she was happy, which was most of the time, and I knew when she was sad, which was not all that often.

Daisy came to know and recognize me. The minute I walked through the front door, she honed in on me and zipped clear across the room at full speed. An unbelievably fast walker at 85, she buzzed around everywhere, although no one knew exactly where she was going. I wondered if even she knew.

Sometimes, when something captured her attention, she stopped and stared, sometimes laughing or smiling. Yet when she saw me, she knew exactly where she was headed, and nothing would distract her.

She reminded me of a sunflower or a pumpkin: bright, sunny and happy, with a warm glow. She had an adorable, round face, with two dimples on her cheeks that came out often because she smiled all the time. Her short, straight hair and bangs framed her face like a picture frame. Always dressed in pastel pinks, blues and yellows, in stretch and cotton knits, she was a tiny lady, not more than five foot tall, with meaty little legs that moved with the speed of a woman half her age.

When she came towards me, she held out her arms, as if carrying an imaginary box, with her blue eyes a little dazed and glassy, yet always holding a smile. She moved in an almost robotic way, as if not quite sure what she would do next.

Every day I greeted her with a hug. "Daisy, Daisy, my beautiful Daisy," I would say in a high-pitched voice filled with exuberant play, shaking my head back and forth, while holding her face between my hands, pressing my nose to her button nose three, four times. Wrinkling up her nose in delight, she giggled like a school girl. Then I gave her a big hug, quickly kissed her forehead and nose several times, and squeezed her cheeks. Smiling endlessly, she would look at me as if I were a long-lost friend. Maybe she thought I was someone else from her past, but that did not matter. What mattered was that she found a friend in me. Hand in hand, we would go walking from one end of the hallway to the other, back and forth, back and forth, my steps keeping up with her quick, short steps.

Daisy never grew tired, or so it seemed. One pleasant spring afternoon, she led me to her room, which looked like a big dollhouse. Her bed was covered with a pink floral spread with ruffles and lace and a collection of stuffed animals sitting cozily on top like old, welcoming friends. Miniature pieces of furniture and porcelain tea sets on top of crocheted doilies were displayed on a mantel. Frilly pillows were scattered around the room on wicker chairs, where her collection of dolls sat amicably, like children at a tea party.

Old dolls with Victorian dresses, new dolls with sunny, cheerful faces that reminded me of Daisy, dolls wearing hats, necklaces, and earrings, some with long, curly, hair, others with short hair, one with red hair that when you pressed the button on her belly, it made her hair grow long or short. I pressed the button to make her hair long, then short, then long, then, short again, deciding that she should have short hair like Daisy. We giggled. She may not have understood words, but she understood fun-loving laughter and smiles.

The warmth in the room came not only from the charming décor, but also from the sunlight streaming in rainbows reflected from crystals hanging in the window in snowflake and heart shapes. Opening the window, I breathed in a flowery scent, luscious and delicious, which I recognized as orange blossoms. It was mixed with moist earth and freshly cut grass.

"Smells so good, Daisy! Just like you. You remind me of spring, a spring that never goes away. Eternal, never growing old, never tiring, just like the Daisy you are. Can you smell the flowers?" I asked, wrinkling my nose with the hope that the gesture would help her to understand. I don't know if she smelled the flowers, but she wrinkled her nose too.

In the distance there were children's voices at play, mixed with their laughter and birdsong that wove with our laughter like a beautiful song of spring, with all the notes blending together harmoniously. I suddenly felt like a child again and remembered one spring day when I played with a favorite doll that resembled one of Daisy's. It wasn't orange blossoms that I smelled then; it was blooming lilacs. Our street was filled with lilac bushes and boysenberry bushes which hung heavy with fruit that I picked and put in a big pot and fed to the doll with her daisy-like face, except her mouth would not open. I kept trying to force them to go in but instead they dribbled down in juicy purple red drops all over her dress.

My mother was not too happy when she saw the doll's stained dress, which she had just sewn, but it did not matter because it was spring. I felt like that child all over again with a heart both innocent and divine as Daisy and I laughed sweet, delicious, bubbly laughter. It felt like we had an unspoken understanding between us of the power and magic of play.

I felt like I was playing in a gigantic doll house, as Daisy and I went hand-in-hand to her display of hats. Her collection hung on hooks: wide floppy hats in an assortment of colors with bows and ribbons, lace, and flowers in a variety of textures such as straw, cotton, velour, and velveteen; little berets in black and red, some extra soft and fuzzy because they were made out of angora. She loved hats. She loved dressing up, and from what I was told, she was quite the social butterfly going out drinking and dancing until late in the evening. She never grew tired then, either.

One by one, I took down her hats, gauging which one she seemed to respond with the most exuberance. "Do you like this one, Daisy?" I asked. "How about this one, or what do you think of this one?" I put back one after another, but when I pulled down a big wide-brimmed powder-blue hat with pink and yellow flowers, her arms reached out for it immediately, as her face lit up.

"You like this one, don't you, Daisy! Let's put this one on!" It looked like an Easter Bonnet. Tapping her nose, I told her that she looked just like an Easter bunny. She liked that and smiled that contagious smile of hers.

Rummaging through her drawer, I picked up a tube of pink lipstick and put it on her curled-up, happy lips. Sparkles of delight replaced the glassy daze in her blue eyes.

"Look, Daisy," I said while pointing to the mirror. She looked with glee at her pink lips and powder-blue hat reflected in the mirror. "You look adorable, but wait one minute, we're still not finished," I said. After finding blush, I brushed it in light, sweeping motions on her cheeks. Without losing her attention, she sat quietly, a remarkable feat. She was focused on the task of being made up to look pretty.

Then I took out a box with her collection of costume jewelry, and together we chose a pair of earrings: big, round pink balls dangling from thin, gold chains. When I put them on, she let out a roaring, purry laugh.

"Look Daisy," I said, "how pretty you look." She liked what she saw, but was getting anxious. I could see that she wanted to get up and go again, to walk again, endlessly walking, but this time ready to show the world what she looked like in her special girlie-girl attire. It was a Friday afternoon, the time for social hour, with music and snacks. It was a lively atmosphere. Still holding hands with Daisy, I shook, wiggled and stepped in time with the music. Smiling, she watched me shake and wiggle again, moving my head from side to side. "Let's dance, Daisy. You do it too! Shake it a little! Come on Daisy, dance with me too."

She moved her head from side to side and then took her first step, wiggling her bottom that was puffy and round from her diaper. Then giving a little shimmy, she moved into a dance with great ease, as if she had done this many times in her life. With Daisy smiling her big, bright, pink lipstick smile that never seemed to fade, we danced for the entire 45 minute program. Daisy's big pink ball earrings dangled and swayed back and forth, up and down, like popcorn popping in a popper; she bobbed her head and wide-brimmed hat in a fun loving spirit, just as she must have done in her younger days.

THE DOLL THAT CHANGED HER LIFE

Essential Points

When with an individual who has Alzheimer's, learn to:

◆ Encourage him to engage in activities he can enjoy and feel successful doing.
◆ Praise small accomplishments.
◆ Allow yourself to play more.
◆ Enter her world, and see through her eyes.
◆ Look for the emotion behind the words or actions.
◆ Be without judgment.

Flo's life suddenly changed with the arrival of a new being -- a plastic, infant-size doll. She found it one day, by chance abandoned on the piano bench in the dining hall. Her life went from dismal to joyous. That doll, with its button nose, pink cheeks, blue eyes, and little mouth puckered in the shape of an O, as if muttering the word *Mama*, birthed new meaning into Flo's lackluster existence. Suddenly, she had a purpose, something to live for each day. She now felt something she had not felt in a long time, love and tenderness. Every day she sat in the same armchair in the hallway, taking care of that plastic baby doll, as if it were her own. Lifting the doll, as if in play, she smiled and giggled, with *coochy, coochy coo* baby talk, shaking her head back and forth, and wrinkling up her nose in delight. Then holding the baby close to her chest, she patted her back gently.

Taking the baby from her chest and tapping her playfully on the nose, she would say, "You're a good little baby, aren't you, aren't you?" while gazing at her adoringly, her eyes filled with such love and joy that I had not seen before.

Before the baby came, Flo was often agitated and confused. Never able to sit still, she always roamed around the hallways, back and forth, up and down, going into other residents' rooms, picking up odd things, like a brush or a watch, a tube of lipstick or a hand-held mirror, sometimes a set of keys, and if anyone tried to take it away, she would get angry and put up a fight, insisting that it was hers. She really believed this.

At times, Flo would wander into an activity, but unable to focus, she would get up and wander around in her own world while the activity was still going on, stumbling into chairs, bumping into other residents. Sometimes, she would go up to the front of the room and make unintelligible utterances to the program leader. Her gray eyes were always cloudy and vacant as she gazed at you, but it felt as if that empty stare went right through you. Sometimes I would take her by the hand and have her sit next to me. Sometimes, she sat quietly, but more often than not, she would get up again and make more unintelligible utterances. If I responded with something based on bits and pieces of what I thought she was saying, my words became other words to her, made to fit within her world, the one she had created. Flo had Alzheimer's and suffered from depression as well, but that doll transformed her life. Now she was a mother, and had a place in the world.

No one could take her little baby away from her, but often other residents tried. They liked the baby and wanted one, too, but Flo would get angry and fight, as if she were fighting for her life, clutching the doll tightly.

One day, there was quite a stir among the residents. Had they not been in wheelchairs, I feared a brawl would have broken out. That day, the baby was *naked*. The doll's one and only dress was being washed, but the residents did not know that. They thought it was indecent that a mother would let her little baby go naked like that. A group of four women congregated in one section of the hallway, whispering to one another, while glaring at Flo.

"What kind of mother is she, who lets her baby go without clothes like that?" one demanded.

"She is immoral," replied the lady next to her, hunched over in her wheelchair.

"The baby should be taken away from her," whispered another, shaking her finger vigorously, like a judge.

"Yes, that's right," the other chimed in, with glasses so thick, it was difficult to see the hard stare she was giving poor Flo. "Teach her a lesson about how to take care of a baby properly."

The whispers soon turned to shouts. The only way the residents were pacified was when I got a little lap blanket to put around the baby.

Whenever Flo was without the doll, be it misplaced or taken, she forgot all about the baby and returned to her agitated and confused wanderings, speaking mumbo jumbo, an empty expression in her eyes. I felt very protective of Flo and the baby, and wondered where the little plastic baby had disappeared. I searched until I found her and brought her to Flo.

"Look, Flo, I found your baby. She was crying because she didn't know where you were. She needs you, Flo. Look at this sweet little baby of yours."

Suddenly, Flo remembered. She remembered her years of being a mother, something that had never left her. She would remember her sweet little coochy coo doll again. Then she would stop her wandering and sit down with the baby. Elation filled her eyes. She was content and at peace again. Her life was birthed again with meaning, as she held the baby in her arms.

"How adorable your little one is," I said to her one day while gazing at the doll, as if she *were* some precious, little being.

Flo smiled proudly while replying, "Isn't she the sweetest little thing you ever did see?"

She held the baby out for me to admire. While I played with the baby, giving her a little *coochy, coochy, coo*, Flo beamed with joy over my praise.

"You are such a good mother, Flo," I said.

"I try, I try my best," she replied.

Her family came in to visit one day and noticed how loving she was with the doll. I told them about how that little doll had changed her life. That made them happy. I told them about the gossip and the brawl that could have broken out about the nakedness of the doll. They laughed, yet took to heart what I said. The next time they came to visit, they brought a whole new set of clothing for the doll!

Flo was tickled. She held up each frilly little item, smiling and saying, "Ah, how precious they all are." It was hard to choose which one she would put on the doll. Finally, deciding on the ruffled pink and white polka dot dress with matching bonnet, she took off the old dress with great tenderness. When she put on the new one, she glowed with the bliss that only a mother knows.

Further thoughts

♦ If your elder has Alzheimer's and suddenly discovers meaning in a plastic doll, validate her. Don't argue that the doll is not real. Allow yourself to PLAY and to see how the doll may be restoring her connection to life by having to care for and love a child. The act of nurturing brings back a purpose in living.

♦ If you are struggling with how to keep your elder engaged, go back to what he or she did for a living? Did it give her meaning? What were his hobbies?

♦ I worked with one 85-year old man who had been a postman for 40 years before retiring twenty years earlier. Dispirited, he wandered about aimlessly. But suddenly his life changed when the Activity Director gave him a big leather mail bag filled with mail and strapped it over his shoulder. Every day she asked him to deliver the mail to the residents and office staff. Now he had a mission. Someone was always with him to make sure the mail was delivered correctly. Bursting with smiles, he was a changed man.

♦ I worked with another elder who used to be a lawyer. We set up a desk for him with his name displayed on a little gold plaque. Above the desk was a sign that advertised free legal counsel. Not only did he keep his mind active, by dipping into his memory for solutions to legal problems, but he also felt he was helping people—and he was. Every day during his designated office hour, he found several residents waiting to see him.

♦ In some cases this approach may not be an alternative. I knew an elder who was once known by her large family as the warmest, kindest person, who was admired for her skills as a homemaker and mother. She loved baking, cooking, raising a family, and taking care of the household. As she reached her seventies, her personality began to change drastically. She became hostile and would fling plates and glasses at family members, as well as bury all of her frying pans and pots in the backyard, never to be seen or used again. She was diagnosed with frontotemperal dementia, which affects personality and behavior. To encourage her to reenact her roles as mother and homemaker would have been inappropriate.

A MIRACULOUS DISCOVERY OF TRIVIA

Essential points

When with someone who has Alzheimer's:

- ♦ Explore and discover what skills or activities he or she will enjoy and feel successful doing.
- ♦ Design activities around those skills.
- ♦ Praise accomplishments.

I was leading a small group in a game of trivia. Jean, a lanky and petite African American woman with cat-shaped glasses and short silver gray hair, stood in the doorway listening intently to each question I asked. Everyone else in the room looked at each other blankly, trying hard to jog their memories for the answers, yet to no avail. Holding her leather bag in one hand, Jean raised the other in the air with verve and declared, "Cairo! The capital of Egypt is Cairo."

I turned my head, baffled by her quick and easy response. It seemed to glide out through her lips, without thought, without having to probe her memory, simply there at the tip of her tongue.

"What is the capital of France?" I asked, but when I saw more of the same puzzled expressions, yet again, I added, "I will give you a hint..." but before I could finish my sentence, Jean, who furrowed her brow as if concentrating, snapped out the word, "Paris, Paris is the capital of France."

"Very good," I replied, stunned.

"The next," she retorted.

Going to the next question, I asked, "What is the capital of Mississippi?"

This time, before I even had a chance to think about a hint or two to give, Jean replied, "Jackson," with a slight, southern twang. She was from Mississippi. "Jackson is the capital," she confirmed while walking into the room, taking a seat at the center, putting her handbag down on the table, as if ready to proceed to the next question. The slump in her posture had suddenly transformed into shoulders back, chin up, body held straight and tall with a dignified confidence. She carried herself with the poise of a scholar.

Jean had been a scholar and once was a university librarian. I was thrilled, silently rooting her on, yet also still completely baffled.

In the six months I had worked with Jean, I had never seen her clear-headed and lucid. She had Alzheimer's, and I was used to seeing her wander from one end of the hall to the other continuously for much of the day. If you spoke to her, she would look at you as if you spoke a language she could not understand.

Other times, she wandered into the activity room, mumbling to herself as if she were in her own world, and whatever we were doing was non-existent or part of another world far removed from her own. She might decide to stay for a few minutes, continuing her private mumblings, then wander back out. On another occasion, she came into the room, gave orders to someone whom no one else could see, while busying herself with moving chairs and various objects to the side, rearranging the room to her liking.

No one thing really held her interest, or at least nothing that I was aware of at that time, until I discovered her incredible memory when it came to facts. Happily, I continued asking questions, and Jean freely rattled off the answers.

How ecstatic I was to discover how to connect with her! I kept rooting her on silently, watching how this game of trivia had completely absorbed her attention. She was there, completely present and alert.

PART XI

SEEING BEYOND THE ANGER

34

ESTHER

Essential points

♦ Look behind the anger.
♦ Listen without judgment.
♦ Provide comfort, understanding, and support.
♦ Know what you can do to help, and what you cannot do.
♦ Take a deep breath, and remain centered and calm.
♦ Know your boundaries and never endanger yourself.

> *If we could read the secret history of our enemies,*
> *we should find in each man's life sorrow and suffering*
> *enough to disarm all hostility.*

> Henry Wadsworth Longfellow

Esther was said to be delusional and a bit crazy. A large and portly woman, she always reminded me of a queen because of her regal and commanding stature. One day she sat in her wheelchair, dressed in her usual colorful flamboyance, with a red silk scarf tied in a big bow around her neck, her silver white hair teased and sprayed into a bouffant, each strand in its proper place. Her diamond stud earrings sparkled against her alabaster face dabbed with rouge and red lipstick.

That day a demure woman in her 90s, her mouth a little puckered without her dentures, returned from the hospital on a stretcher. When my co-worker and I rushed up to welcome her home, she smiled sweetly at us.

Esther glared at the innocent lady propped up in the stretcher, raised her right arm, as if giving a command and bellowed, "This woman is a fraud, take her away, she doesn't belong here." Everyone in the hallway — staff, residents in wheelchairs and visitors alike — was electrified by this rippling surge of energy and paused from what they were doing to view the spectacle. Though everything came to a standstill, no one uttered a word.

Roiled that no one responded, Esther bellowed again, "Take her away, she is a fraud, did you hear me, I tell you she is a fraud, don't let her fool you, she is a fraud and doesn't belong here, take her away now!"

The returning lady, unable to hear without her hearing aids, cocked her head in bewilderment and looked at Esther. Shaking her head, my co-worker looked at me and chuckled. I was equally as amused.

We had seen this kind of thing from Esther before. I looked over at the young man wheeling the stretcher who looked as if at any moment his smile would turn into a peal of laugher, as he wheeled his patient down the hall and into her room.

Maybe Esther was a little crazy, a little delusional. She could be difficult. Sometimes when I came to work, the minute I walked through the doors of skilled nursing, I could hear her shouting in an almost delirious rage. Most of the time she was taken to her room where the door was shut, and she was given medication.

My initial response to Esther's anger was like everyone else's, to walk away. But as I got to know and understand her better,

I could not walk away without attempting some sort of conciliation. After seeing the wounded spirit behind the craziness and the rage, I wanted in some small way to help. I didn't mean to solve her problems, but just to be there for her, to listen and, if possible, to help bring more peace into her heart.

Esther had other facets to her personality. She was lively, witty, well-read and extremely intelligent, an interesting woman with many fascinating stories of her travels around the world. She could also be incredibly loving and caring.

The first time I saw this side of Esther, a new resident had moved into a room down the hall from her. The newcomer was a gentle and kind lady in her early 90s. Hearty and stout, with bright, blue eyes and silver hair, she was an attractive, older woman, with rosy cheeks and only a few wrinkles. She also had dementia and when she tried to speak, a few jumbled words tumbled out. Often she sat in her wheelchair with her hands folded together in her lap, nodding and smiling.

Her name was Eva, and whenever Esther saw her, she would adoringly caress Eva's forehead and hair, then hold her age-spotted hand, while telling her how much she cared about her and promising to look after her. "I will never let anything bad happen to you," Esther would say, while Eva repeatedly smiled and nodded.

Esther sat with Eva every day. When she did not see Eva in the hallway, Ester sought her out. Wheeling herself down the hall, she called for her friend, except the name she used was not Eva.

"Miriam, where are you?" she would call, wheeling more frantically and hurriedly as time passed without hearing Eva reply.

"Miriam, Miriam, where are you?" Going into Eva's room, she would look for her in her bed that usually was empty. Eva had a family that she went out with from time to time. She also had doctors' visits and other appointments to keep.

"Where did you take her?" Esther would shout at the nurses' station with clenched fists, as if ready to do battle.

"Esther, please calm down, Eva is out with her family," a nurse replied.

"You are lying, I know you are lying. You cannot fool me. You've taken her away, haven't you?"

"Calm down Esther, Eva will be back. She went out with her family."

Convinced that the nurse was lying, Esther continued to rage in her bellowing voice.

"Look what they have done. They have taken her away, and now they are lying."

Not knowing what else to do, the nurses often gave her medication, which was not an easy task because Esther fought them. Then, against her will, she would be taken to her room, where she continued to yell until the medication took effect — that is, if she acquiesced to taking the medicine.

What no one knew then, including myself, was that Esther once had a sister whose name was Miriam. Whenever she saw Eva, Esther saw the sister she loved and cared about deeply, who was taken away and put into an insane asylum as a teenager. One of Esther's friends shared this with me, and from that day forward, my relationship with Ester would never be the same.

That story touched me deeply, especially after seeing how tender she could be with Eva. My perception of Esther shifted. Under the crazed, angry woman, I saw her wounded brokenness. Poignantly, I felt her brokenness, with its sharp edges, piercing me in a strangely familiar and tender way. I, too, have been wounded. I, too, have been broken.

One day, when Esther was brought to her room in one of her delirious rages, I slipped in to see her. I told her how sorry I was that she had to suffer like this. After some time of listening to her scream and yell about how they are all lying, how they have taken "Miriam" away, I asked her about her sister. She wheeled herself to the chest of drawers that was covered with framed pictures. There were several pictures of her and her husband, who had passed away 15 years ago, as well as a couple of old black and whites of a young woman who resembled Esther. She picked up one of those affectionately, holding it for a few minutes with the same tenderness in her eyes that I saw when she was with Eva.

"This is my sister," she said. The girl was a plump teenager, with a round cherub face and a dimple in her chin, just like Esther's, with curly, brunette hair. Sitting on a cozy Victorian style chair, she held a little black dog curled in her lap.

"She wasn't crazy, like my father said. She was bold and outspoken. My father didn't like that. He thought a woman should be docile, subservient, and silent. He called her mad, and right in front of me, he would beat her with a big leather strap until she was bleeding and black and blue all over." A tear fell from the corner of Esther's eye, an emotion I hadn't seen in her before. I got a tissue for her as more tears fell.

"It made me angry! I was always the quiet one, the one who didn't speak much, because I was afraid of my father, but when I saw that he was taking her away to the crazy house, I couldn't be quiet any more. Never would I allow anyone to hurt my sister like that again. Never would I be silent. I became the tough girl at school, you know, the kind everyone was afraid of, yet if you were my good friend, I'd be yours for life, I'd take good care of you and not let anything bad happen to you."

"I wish you had been my friend when I was growing up." I said. "I was one of those scrawny little kids that cried a lot and was always picked on by the bigger girls. I know you would have taken care of them for me, Esther."

"You better believe I would, darling," she replied.

While Esther continued sharing with me, I began to realize that she felt responsible for what had happened. She felt like she could have stopped it had she not been so afraid of her father, and had she spoken out. I understood what she felt because when I was four years old, my father died, and not really understanding death, only that he was gone and would not come back, I felt like I was responsible, like I had done something wrong that caused his departure, and that was the reason he was not coming back, so I understood how Esther might have felt. That story played over and over in her mind, causing her so much torment and grief, and it festered. It was as if through Eva she could change her destiny by doing it differently this time, undo what had been done.

The more I got to know Esther, the more I loved her. She loved old movies and liked to tell me about all the movies she had seen, who the stars were, and what was happening at that time in her life and in world history. Her memory was impeccable. I also enjoyed listening to her stories of her world travels with her husband, to whom she was married for nearly 50 years. During her fascinating life, her husband's work had taken them to Africa, Japan, and India.

While I was planning my trip to India, I talked with her often about it. As happy as she seemed to be for me as she described all the magnificent places there were to see, I always sensed a bit of sadness and agitation, as if she were disturbed by something, not something I said or did, but something else.

One day, during a conversation about India, she became so pale, with her lips purplish and dry, as if she were about to faint. She shook her head back and forth nervously and repeated, "Be careful, darling, be careful, be careful, please do be careful when you are there. You know things are much different there." It was as if she were speaking in the present, yet her eyes reflected another time, another place, when she was in India 15 years earlier. Though India was a land she had loved and found fascinating, it left a haunting memory.

She then shared the story of how her husband had suddenly taken ill in India.

"Violently ill," she said, shaking her head, her tear-filled eyes gazing into the distance, "so violently ill. You cannot imagine. We didn't know what to do, what it was caused from. He was too sick even to go see a doctor. I called for one to come. After examining him for all the usual diseases, the doctor could not give him a diagnosis. It could be something he ate, the doctor said. Is there a chance of recovery? I asked. Only time will tell, he replied. Time only made him sicker, so we brought him to the hospital. No one could say what was wrong, but my husband knew he was dying. He made peace with it, but I could not. I did not want to believe it. I called for a rabbi. I found one in the nearest city. It was a day's journey by train, but he made it there just before my husband took his last breath. I couldn't do a thing. I couldn't think straight. I couldn't act. I had someone from home come and help me. We brought the body back. My friends and family were all waiting, but what could I do? What could I tell them? They wanted me to do shiva,* yet I couldn't even do that. I was not prepared to accept his passing."

Esther broke down, sobbing.

Tears can heal and sooth, tears can transform, tears are like a balm that washes the grief away. I held her while she wept. I will never forget that moment, nor the stories that she shared with me. Nor will I forget the tenderness I suddenly felt for her upon learning the story of her sister, discovering the other face behind the rage.

I also came to discover that sometimes it simply was not possible to reach out to Esther and get through. Sometimes she became so enraged and delirious that in her mind even those who were kind and loving to her were conspiring against her. It was then that I had to walk away because there was no other choice. You cannot change someone. You cannot make someone respond.

In spite of those times, I never stopped loving her. One day, I told her how she was always in my prayers. She thanked me and said, "Keep praying for me, I need all the prayers I can get, darling."

Two months after I stopped working at that community, I kept thinking about her. During my morning meditation, I kept seeing her face appear to me so vividly and clearly, almost as if she were there. That week, I kept sending her thoughts of peace and love. Something in me told me to call the community, just to see how she was. I was told that she had passed away that very week. Truly, I hope she found the peace within herself that she so needed.

* Shiva – a seven day period of morning after someone's death, where relatives and friends visit to offer support to the family of the deceased.

EVERY WOMAN'S HERO

Essential points

♦ Learn to listen to the same story again and again, as if it were the first time.
♦ Support and celebrate the stories your elders share about their life journey.

Miriam was *every woman's hero,* or at least that was how I saw her and what I called her after she finished telling me a story she would tell me over and over again. I did not mind. Every time she told this important story, it was with the same dramatic expression, flooded with great emotion.

Often Miriam sat quietly in her wheelchair with a book in her lap, her reading glasses pivoted at the tip of her nose, her feet firmly implanted on the ground, with a sturdy earthiness like an earth mother.

Crouching down next to her, I would ask about the book she was reading.

Patting me on the cheek, she would say, "You are such a dear girl," while setting her book down, taking her glasses off, and our conversation would begin. Somehow all our conversations led to that same story, which Miriam always told it as if for the first time, forgetting that I had heard it several times before.

"Can you imagine, I lived during a time when women were forbidden what men were always entitled to? All I wanted was to get an education!" she exclaimed, indignant over the injustice of her time. Clenching her hand into a fist, she would raise her arm boldly, dauntlessly, declaring her truth proudly to the world, a truth she was determined to fight for and win through justice. This story had marked her life, forging the path of her highest calling – to learn and teach.

Miriam lived during a time when it was not easy for a woman to make choices and pursue them freely, like getting an education and having a career. In Miriam's family, it was unthinkable because her very stern and strict father insisted that it is the man who makes all the decisions in the house.

In his view, women should not be allowed an education. That was the exclusive domain of men. Women were supposed to stay home, take care of the house and raise a family. That was their sole function. This view did not stop Miriam from pursuing her dream. She was relentless ever since childhood, when her great love of books and learning all began. "I was determined," she said, "I wouldn't let my father or anyone else stop me."

Her gentler and kinder mother saw that side of Miriam and wanted to support her dream, so mother and daughter colluded in pursuing the vision. Any extra money the mother had, she gave to Miriam to put aside for her education. Unbeknownst to her father, Miriam got a job and worked after school, saving all her money until she had enough to pay for her college tuition. Throughout college, she studied during the day and worked in the evening.

As Miriam was busy developing her mind, her father had another plan for her. He saw that she was coming of age, and it was time for her to get married and raise a family. She did not want that, or at least not then. Against her father's wishes, she refused the men he chose, while continuing her education until she finished. Then she saw her dream blossom. She became a teacher and moved out of the house to live on her own.

At that point in the telling of her story, any bitterness that may have been there diminished, and her slumped body became more erect. Her blue eyes emanated a joyous strength and willful determination as she remembered how she had lived her dream and accomplished it on her own. For that, she was proud. Eventually, she did marry, but only after she had taught for a few years.

"In those days," she told me, "you had to be single to teach. A woman was not allowed to teach if she was married, so I had to give up my post." When she got married, she did not see that as a defeat. Her new ambition was to raise her daughters, giving them what she was not given so easily, and to teach them what she had not been taught — that women have the freedom to choose, and the importance of developing their minds.

"I raised three beautiful daughters, and their education was always number one. Whatever they wanted, I gave them."

In many ways, her daughters continued living her dreams. They were all high achievers, with brilliant minds and careers, yet still raised families.

Miriam often raised her hands and exclaimed, "Men! Who needs them? They only get in the way! Women could live perfectly fine lives without men!"

Whenever I see Rosie the Riveter, I think of Miriam, because she is just like Rosie, with her flexed arm held high in determination, ready to transform the world by changing how the world thinks of women.

Often during activities, Miriam got riled if anything ever came up in the news or in a program involving injustices done toward women. She would shake her fists and let you know exactly what she thought. She was not afraid of speaking out.

Maybe, there was one thing at one time that she *would* have been afraid to declare openly to the world. *Maybe*. To have done so, would have been anathema. Her daughter once told me that, had Miriam been born at a later time, she probably would have been a lesbian. "My mother! She has no need for men!" We both laughed.

One day, I saw an article in *Newsweek* written by an 81-year-old woman who had been a lesbian her whole life but had never been able to say this openly before then. Strictly forbidden during her younger days, everything had to be kept secret. But times were changing and she could declare her truth to the world for the first time, *in a big way*, by publishing an article in *Newsweek*. She spoke about her difficulties, and how now, with same sex marriage being legal in some states, she was coming out, with pride.

Inspired by that article, I clipped it out with Miriam in mind, and read it in one of my daily news programs, which she liked to attend. When I finished reading the article, I looked over at Miriam. Applauding this woman's bold and liberating stance, Miriam exclaimed, "She was finally able to declare her truth to the world. I think that is marvelous! What a fine woman!"

PART XIII

WHEN THE SUN GOES DOWN

36

A BEATIFIC VISION

Essential points

When with someone who has dementia:

- Enter his or her world, as long as no one is endangered.
- Be present, without judgment.

While I sat at the dining table conversing with Dorothy, a lovely resident who once was a doctor, we admired the nuances in the sky, moving, shifting, passing with the blink of an eye as colors deepened in shades of indigo and golden orange, puffed up like pregnant penguins' bellies, swirling around and around in a mysterious glow of some bigger presence.

"Lovely, lovely," she said, "isn't it? Looks like it might rain tomorrow."

"Yes," I said, while we paused silently.

Silverware clinked against plates and voices carried on in other conversations, with caregivers feeding, while more plates were brought in and taken out, when all of a sudden, Virginia, sitting at the far end of the table, put down her fork, stood up from the table, lifted her arms and exclaimed in her proper British accent, "Oh my, oh my, oh my," her voice deepening with each *oh my* into a sultry growl. She pressed her hands to her chest, as if admiring something stunning.

"Oh my, oh my," she continued, "just look at him, just look, he has come to get me." She shook her head slowly, as if in awe of the beauty before her eyes. "Oh my, just look at him, isn't he beautiful?"

With her hot pink, furry slippers flopping away, she walked over to the window and pressed her hand to the glass, her eyes agog and exclaimed, "Oh yes, there he is! My man, oh yes, and he is all mine!"

Conversation came to a standstill, while Dorothy and I looked at one another amused. I could almost read her thoughts because they were mine as well. *What was Virginia up to now? Could it be possible the sunset was him, her man? Maybe. Anything was possible.*

"No, I don't think so," Dorothy declared, with her arthritic hand held up to her mouth, chuckling.

We both knew Virginia. She had been the proper English woman her whole life, but now that she was older, she was letting go of that old, worn-out skin which no longer suited her. Now her life was about MEN, whenever and wherever one could be found. There were few male residents and workers in skilled nursing, and whenever one came around, she batted her eyes and smiled... She followed the man everywhere, and if he sat down to lead an activity, she would plop herself next to him, fondle his hair, caress his back, and stare at him adoringly.

I got up from the table, went over to Virginia and asked, "What is it, Virginia? Where is your man?"

"He is right over there." I looked but did not see anything. "Where?" I asked.

"Look, right there," she replied, pointing to the corner ledge of the balcony, where a pigeon stood with plumped-up feathers and head turned around in the midst of grooming himself.

"Oh my, isn't he gorgeous, isn't he the most beautiful thing you ever did see? And he is my man, all mine! Look at his bow tie and suit: so elegant, so regal, so fine!" she gushed, with her hands clasped together against her chest. "Yes, he certainly is, isn't he?"

I threw my arms around her and replied, "Yes, yes, Virginia, he certainly is beautiful."

We continued admiring the pigeon, while everyone else went back to their conversations and dining. Dorothy chuckled, "Oh my, oh my, what a funny place this is!"

TWO STRANGERS NO LONGER ALONE

Essential points

When with individuals who have dementia:

♦ Validate their world, if it provides comfort and is causing no harm.
♦ Learn to let go of your notions of reality and see theirs without judgment.
♦ Learn to see humor and grace.

"What is all *that* ruckus?" I asked the charge nurse, a buxom, middle-aged Nigerian woman, as she sorted medicines into little paper cups on her medicine cart. Her ears perked and she smiled prankishly while listening to all the shuffling sounds, clinking, clanking, chinking, metal upon metal, a sliding screech on tiles in the midst of muffled voices. "What is *all that* noise?" I asked again.

"Could be anything at this time of day," she replied, pointing to the open door of the shower room that was also used as a storage area for things like old wheelchairs and walkers. "There! That is exactly where it is coming from!"

In the shower room, we discovered Edie and Lucy, who decided *this* was their home, and *it was their* job was to rearrange, decorate, cozy up and make it as comfortable as possible.

The charge nurse and I smiled playfully while watching Lucy give instructions to Edie on how and where to move each walker, each wheelchair. Neither of us could understand their language with its nonsensical conjugation of sentences, yet each responded to the other. Lucy's body language told us that she was the boss, giving instructions, and Edie understood.

"What are you ladies doing in here?" I asked. Edie looked up from the walker she was rolling over to Lucy, who took it, lifted it and set it down in line with another.

"Good, good," Lucy said to Edie.

"Soon we'll be there," Edie replied.

"What are you two ladies doing in here?" the charge nurse asked, repeating my unanswered question.

"We're fixing up our room for the night," Edie replied, while continuing to roll another walker to Lucy, who picked it up again and placed it down in line with the others.

They *really* were making this their home. We may not have understood their gibberish, but they did. Maybe they did not need words and sentences, as we know and use them. Maybe it would have only gotten in the way, as language sometimes does. The body may say more. The heart may say more, and maybe they understood something at a deeper level, like the most simple and basic things that one craves and needs – love, shelter, warmth and friendship.

Lucy and Edie were no longer alone in the world. They had found each other and now they had a shared mission to make this place their own. I could not help wondering *what* this could be, all these wheelchairs lined side by side: *a bed, a night table, a chest?* They somehow were figuring all that out. We certainly could not.

38

BENNY'S ADVENTURE

Essential points

If an individual has Alzheimer's:

♦ Display objects that spark interest, and keep him or her occupied.
♦ Create a safe living space that is pleasant and Alzheimer's friendly.

"Where's Benny? What do you mean you don't know where Benny is? He is always with you!" the charge nurse cried anxiously. It was already dinner, and Benny could not be found, which was rare, because Benny followed me everywhere, without ever saying a word because he had lost the ability to speak.

He had disappeared when I slipped into the ladies' room for a few minutes. At the time, I didn't think anything of it; now I had no idea where he was.

A plump, jolly fellow, balding at the crown, with brown bubble eyes that gazed with zealous enthusiasm, I don't ever remember Benny not smiling. He had a face you could not help but love. I always wanted to tap his nose, pinch his cheeks and say, *you are just the sweetest, most adorable man.*

Once I played catch with him with a big red beach ball. When I tossed it to him, he was not quite sure what to do with it, so he decided the best thing was to hold it tightly against his chest. With that ball, he followed me for the rest of the day.

So this was strange that Benny was nowhere to be found. There was great concern in the air. *Where could he possibly be?* Benny had Alzheimer's, and the day was losing its light. Any moment darkness would come, and still no Benny.

When I returned the following afternoon, I saw Benny roaming around in his usual way. The charge nurse told me what had happened, "I will never know *how* he managed to get out of one of the doors without the alarms going off, but he somehow did."

Benny was a good walker who had been a mailman most of his life. Apparently, he walked down the street, and saw an open garage with walls covered with hanging tools of every kind. Sparked with interest, he went inside, pulled down the tools, and studied them. Perhaps he remembered them, having once held these very objects in his hands.

I wondered what passed through his mind. My guess was that they seemed so familiar to him, yet so strange. *What were they exactly?*, he might have thought, his thought holding a different shape from how we usually think, perhaps a thought without words, more like a hunch or a feeling, a connection attached to a vague memory of having done this before.

What to do with these objects now might have been another question. His hands remembered them well, because he had been a handyman in his spare time. His wife once told me he loved tools and fixing things that would have otherwise been discarded.

I don't know exactly how Benny responded when he was discovered by the homeowner who drove up in his car and saw a stranger fondling his tools. I can only imagine that he probably would have grinned charmingly while gazing with wonder at the man. The man probably figured that Benny was no thief.

In fact, he probably sensed that Benny was harmless and lived at the skilled nursing residence at the top of the hill.

When the man called to notify the residence of an elder in his garage, the charge nurse immediately knew that it was Benny. "Thank god, thank god, that he is all right," she exclaimed. Immediately, Benny was escorted back safely to his home up the street.

Further thoughts

For some delightfully creative approaches to making the living space safe for someone living with Alzheimer's, please see Joanne Koenig Coste's book *Learning to Speak Alzheimer's*.

Some of her suggestions are:

♦ Paint or wallpaper entry doors the same color as the wall, making it harder to see.

♦ Place the functioning lock or doorknob higher or down much lower on the door.

♦ Place a black mat inside the front door to suggest a dark chasm. This will deter your loved one from wandering off into danger.

CHAPTER

39

TELEVISION AND ALZHEIMER'S:
WHAT IS REAL, WHAT IS NOT?

Essential points

If someone has Alzheimer's:

♦ Create an environment conducive to peace and equanimity.
♦ Be mindful of too much violence and conflict on television and in movies.
♦ Provide a sense of purpose in doing a task—and the task will follow.

> *Affirm life, love, unity, and beauty — and stay away from the rest.*

Bennett was an elegant, graceful, and dignified man who lived in a small care residence. He was a successful architect and painter with a lifelong fascination with the Mayan civilization. He loved birds, old clocks, and building model airplanes. Often he sat in the living room in the same chair, his hands folded quietly in his lap, his legs crossed, and while his shoulders slumped a bit from age, his head was always held high.

We often looked at and talked about books with pictures of Mayan ruins, colorful birds, art, photography, or architecture from around the world. Even as Bennet declined in his Alzheimer's, he still had moments when his wit and brilliance shined. He made me laugh and sometimes uttered little pearls of wisdom in the midst of jumbled up words and sentences.

Once while looking at a book about birds, he paused and said, "I wonder why God made so many different varieties of birds. I think we should have a conversation with God about this." Though he no longer built airplanes because it reminded him too much what he couldn't do, I discovered how to encourage him to work on a project with me. When I asked him if he wanted to build a model airplane, he very clearly said no. Then I asked if he would *help me* make one.

"There has to be a purpose," he said.

"What would give you a purpose?"

"If you were doing it because you thought I wanted you to, there wouldn't be a purpose. But if you were doing it because you wanted to, that would be a purpose."

"Good, because I want to build an airplane and need your help."

Likewise, if I asked him if he wanted to paint or draw, he would say no. But if I asked him to *help me make something*, and said I needed his guidance, he would say yes because it gave him a sense of purpose. I asked him for his opinion on colors, lines, shapes, and placement of things while I was drawing. Throughout the process he remained engaged. And his suggestions always made the drawing better.

One day while working on an art project together, I made a mistake and didn't know what to do. My intention was to cut one origami snowflake from a piece of folded paper, but I cut too much from the paper, so instead of it being one piece, it fell into several pieces. I couldn't start all over again because I ran out of paper. When I shared my dilemma with Bennett, he pointed out the fallen scraps of paper and suggested that we do something with them.

It was the perfect solution! Delightedly, I let Bennett know that he solved the problem and that I was so thankful for his suggestion that taught me something about design.

Bennett was a bright spot in my day. I always looked forward to seeing him, but when I visited him one afternoon and knelt down to greet him as he sat in the TV-living room, he didn't respond with the usual smile or warm sparkle in his eyes. He was agitated, restless, fearful, and almost on the verge of tears. When I asked if he wanted to visit in his room as we normally did because it was quieter, he said he could not leave because he had to appear in court and could not get out of it. He was being tried for a crime he didn't commit. Shaken to the core, he said, "How could they do this to a poor old man? They are going to take all my money away and I'll have nothing left."

No matter what I did or said, I couldn't bring the kind of comfort and peace I was hoping for. And when I saw what was on the television--an afternoon court show--I became upset because this could have been prevented. I spoke with the social worker, who was also very upset by this, and then she spoke with the director. The following week, though that show was not on, a movie was playing with a court room scene with a menacing judge.

It was the same sad scenario all over again. I tried to be a consoling presence, but nothing seemed to work until I brought out some essential oils and massage lotion. I asked Bennett to smell the lavender and other scents and then massaged his hands. It worked. He was calm and cheerful again. Although this was highly effective, it would have been infinitely better to be pro-active and preventative by selecting programs that are free from any violence and disturbing conflict.

Further thoughts

Imagine what it would be like if you were being summoned to court for a crime you didn't commit and part of the punishment was that all your hard earned money was going be taken away and you'd have to spend the rest of your days in jail. Pretty horrifying; isn't it?

People with Alzheimer's may not be able to distinguish between what is real and what is not. Be mindful of the kinds of programs they watch. Monitor to see how they respond. If they become anxious and fearful every time they watch a particular program, stop playing it. If you cannot turn the program off because other residents want to watch it, be sure to take them away from the program and occupy them with something else more uplifting.

Suggestions for creating engaging and inspiring activities

♦ Create a calming space that brings healing, peace, and equanimity, especially before bedtime. TV news is *never* a good idea. I've been to some facilities where the news is constantly on. When you are able, put on something else that is more life affirming, or shut off the TV.

♦ Soothing music, nature videos, and CD's can effectively prepare them for a night of restful sleep. CD's with babies or animals playing (please, no violence or hunting) can also be a nice way to end the evening.

♦ The essential oil lavender has calming effects.

♦ Try reframing how you ask someone to work on an art project with you. Change the question from "Do you want to make something?" to "Will you help me make something? I need your help." Ask for their guidance. Ask if they will teach you. Helping others gives a sense of purpose. We all need a purpose in living.

PART XIII

IN THE END, IT'S ALL ABOUT LOVE AND ONLY LOVE

A DEEPER UNDERSTANDING BEYOND WORDS

Essential points

♦ Allow those you care for to care for and comfort you. Caring for someone or something is essential to our nature. It gives purpose and meaning.

♦ Provide more opportunities for your elders to help you.

♦ Don't underestimate someone's capabilities, no matter how much they've lost through illness. Always see the highest and best in them.

♦ Aspire to bring more healing and peace into their world through understanding, empathy, love, wisdom, and kindness.

♦ Don't impose your will. Allow your elders to exercise their right to choose.

> *But, listen to me: for one moment,*
> *quit being sad. Hear blessings*
> *dropping their blossoms*
> *around you. God.*

Rumi

What I remember most of all about Pearl was her eyes. They reminded me of cat's eyes — deep, green, speckled with gold. Like a cat, Pearl could stare with mysterious intensity, as if she knew secrets about you that you yourself did not know, as if she knew exactly what you were thinking, what was hidden in your heart.

You could not fool Pearl. Her wisdom and understanding went beyond the average ken, although she suffered from vascular dementia after a stroke. She also lost her range of motion on one side of her body, as well as the ability to turn her neck to the side, so whenever I talked with her, her eyes moved toward me, which added to her mystery. Then her torso followed, slowly and only partially.

Pearl was an attractive, strong-willed, woman who was fond of wearing red and other bold and bright colors. A woman with her own mind she refused to let anyone tell her how to do something or when to do it, and she absolutely hated the daily prodding that went on at seven o' clock in the morning. She would yell and fight until she got her way.

Who could blame her? She had always gotten up late in the morning. She had worked as a full-time nurse, the 3-11 shift, most of her working life, and *after all, shouldn't it be her prerogative when to get up in the mornings?* She was paying a lot of money to be in skilled nursing, and she wanted to be allowed certain things, like more control over her life and her schedule.

After a few months, her family decided to hire a private duty caregiver who would come every day and let her go to sleep and wake up when she wanted, who would make sure she was showered daily and had her hair and nails done and her face made up. She liked being well dressed and wanted a caregiver who would take the time to do it the way she wanted. She liked dressing in scarves, hats, silk blouses and dresses. Having her own caregiver gave her freedom. It also gave her a sense of dignity.

At times, Pearl could seem perfectly lucid, but after a few minutes something would shift. Her sentences came out fragmented, words got jumbled, and what began as a lucid conversation would fade into empty space, as if all were forgotten. Then, starting another conversation about something entirely different, she would repeat the same process over and over again. Both Pearl's short-term and long-term memory were severely impaired. She could not remember what happened an hour ago, much less the day before, yet I often felt that she remembered something poignant from her past. It was as if she were trying to grasp that memory in order to make sense of it, then all of a sudden it would slip away. Those memories reminded me of a forest shrouded by a dense fog, with one tree that she kept trying to navigate her way to, but each time she lost her bearing, with the fog obscuring her vision, leaving her frustrated, confused, and lost.

Something dark and deep troubled her, pressing down on her. Often she talked about the mistakes that were made in her marriage, a difficult and troubled relationship that lasted for many years. At one time she must have liked to drink, because while sitting next to the table, she would reach for a martini glass and drink from it with the grace and elegance of a sophisticated woman during cocktail hour, yet there was no glass there at all. After a few long slow sips she would say, "I'll have another."

I asked her once what she was drinking. "Gin martini with two olives straight up," she replied in earnest. Not once did I tell her otherwise. It seemed to bring her a sense of security and consolation.

I sat and listened to her while she had her martinis. If I or anyone else were not there, she would still have her martinis while conversing about things past. My deepest wish was that she would make peace with whatever was troubling her and that I would be able to touch her heart in some way that would help to facilitate that peace.

There was a depth to my connection with Pearl that went beyond my understanding. I realized that what I deeply wished for her, she also wished for me. I loved the Pearl she once was whom I learned about through her daughter, as well as the Pearl I knew in the present, who would forget things from one moment to the next.

One day, I came to work troubled and sad. Although on the surface I appeared happy, internally I was weeping and in despair. Typically, I will not let my personal life interfere with my work, and I'm pretty good at it. I go to work, do whatever needs to be done and stay focused on the task.

That day, as always, after the residents had eaten dinner and were brought back from the dining room into the hallway to sit and congregate before bed, I made my rounds and said goodbye to everyone. As I was about to leave, Pearl looked at me with her intense green cat's eyes speckled with gold, her neck half turned, the rest of her body held stiff and said, "Come here, dear."

I knelt down by the wheelchair in front of her. Looking directly into my eyes, she took her hands and put them around the back of my head as she stroked my hair lovingly and asked, "What is it, dear? What is bothering you?"

Totally surprised and touched by her concern, I exclaimed, "Oh Pearl," while giving her a hug.

"What is it, dear? Tell me. I'm here for you," she responded.

I did not know what to say and fell silent, with my hands on her knees, taking in the mysterious beauty of her eyes. Her gaze hypnotized me, and I smiled.

"If I could only do something to lift the pain in your heart," she said, holding my head tenderly. Silence filled that moment — a silence that was full and alive. My smile remained, as if frozen, but my eyes welled with tears, because I felt so touched by her kind and lucid gesture.

Breaking the silence, I said, "You just did, Pearl, you just did by your words and your kindness alone."

"Good, I am glad, dear," she replied. "You know I would do anything for you."

After kissing her and saying goodbye, I walked away feeling truly lighter, freer. I felt lifted by her, with the sadness in my heart transformed into beauty, peace, and light. How grateful I was to know her. She did the very thing I had always wished I could do for her.

The following day when I went to work, Pearl was sitting in the doorway of her room. When she saw me, she called me over and asked, "Are you feeling better today, dear?"

"Yes, Pearl, I *am* feeling better, thanks to you. I only wish that I could give to you what you have given me."

And she said, "Oh you have, dear, you have given more than you will ever know."

Further thoughts

Recently I saw an elder tucked away in the corner of a room sitting in a wheelchair repeating, "All I want to do is help. Let me help you." How true! We all want to feel as if we are helping or caring for something or someone, contributing to some bigger cause outside of ourselves.

Suggestions for creating meaningful and engaging activities:

♦ Ask what causes your elders would like to support and then design activities that contribute to those causes.

Some examples are:

- Providing food for a homeless shelter.

- Knitting hats for women with breast cancer.

- Making blankets, stuffed dolls or animals for children on hospice.

- Fostering a small animal in need of a home.

IF ONLY WE ALL GAVE LOVE LIKE EMMA

Essential Points

When visiting someone with Alzheimer's learn to:

♦ Leave worries and stress at home.
♦ Bring joy and a light heart.
♦ See without judgment.
♦ Look for the emotion behind the words.
♦ Praise small accomplishments.
♦ Don't criticize what she cannot do.
♦ Read stories with an uplifting message more often.

> *Come out of the circle of time*
> *and into the circle of Love.*
>
> —Rumi

With her arms open in a ready-to-embrace gesture, she scuttles toward me spryly, as she always does, as if I were some good friend she has known for years, yet I hardly know her. She always greets me with a big smile and a few kind words of "I love you,

you are so wonderful." Something fey about her enchants and reminds me of a leprechaun. Perhaps it is the sparkle in her aquamarine eyes that are always so round and open as if she were captivated by something she sees.

When I first met Emma, I was doing a storytelling program in assisted living, and it was one of those days when every story fell flat. One elder fell asleep; another couldn't sit still and fidgeted with her handbag, then fumbled nosily through papers; another got up to leave because she was confused and thought this was supposed to be another program; another resident came in late in a disruptive way, decided she did not want to be there after all and left in the same disruptive manner.

Yet I continued reading with enthusiasm, hoping that *this one* would be *the one* that would change the mood, but my hopes were in vain. Or at least not until a story later when I was in the midst of its telling, when a couple walked in discreetly, or at least the husband was trying to be discreet. His wife, Emma, seemed confused about where she was, or what they were doing, and kept asking him what she should do. When she noticed that he was motioning for her to sit down, she took a seat. Graciously, her husband apologized for the disruption, although it did not bother me, and I welcomed them both. He was a sweet, kind-looking man, and she was a bubbly, always happy, and smiling woman with Alzheimer's and once she was seated, she listened quietly and attentively.

What went through her mind as she listened? Did the words make sense to her? Did the story reach out and touch her in some way? Maybe she understood something on a level that was hidden from us. Maybe she sensed my enthusiasm and good intentions. Or maybe she had no clue where she was or why she was there, but realized that this was the way to behave in this situation.

Whatever the reason, the story held her attention, and when I finished, she blew kisses at me, as if I were a star in some grand theatre, clapping her hands with vigor and exclaiming, "That was wonderful, wonderful, wonderful! Thank you! I love you!"

Inspired by her enthusiastic response, I read the next story. With the same attention, she listened, and when I finished, she clapped her hands again with the same gusto. I told more stories. Each time she responded with the same zest, clapping her hands and exclaiming, "That was wonderful! Thank you! I love you!"

Two ladies glared at Emma each time she uttered a word. One yelled at Emma's husband, "She always causes a disruption! She doesn't belong here! You know better than to bring her here."

Her friend chimed in, "She should be taken out! She belongs on the other unit, not here!" Then turning to me, her fingers making circular motions by the side of her head, she rolled her eyes and said, "She has a few screws loose."

"It's O.K.," I responded. "She has a right to be here and she is not bothering anyone."

"Well! If that is how you feel!" she replied, indignantly. After thanking everyone for coming, I went over to thank Emma for her enthusiasm. "You are wonderful," she exclaimed, "and I love you!"

"I love you too!" I replied, "I am happy that you came." I introduced myself to her and her husband. Emma continued smiling and repeating, "I love you! You are so wonderful!"

"And you are wonderful, too!" I said.

Emma reached for me and gave me a hug.

Her husband apologized and said, "I am sorry she is like that! I hope she did not cause you any disturbance." Later, I discovered that Emma's husband was just as sweet and kind as he looked. The staff had suggested on a number of occasions that Emma be put in the Alzheimer's unit, saying it was too much for him, but he insisted on taking care of her himself, and he did a wonderful job.

"Not at all," I replied. "There is nothing to be sorry about. She didn't do anything wrong. I am only too happy to have met you both."

"Oh yes," she repeated. "Thank you, thank you, thank you, it was so wonderful and you are wonderful! I love you."

"I love you too. You are wonderful!" I replied.

Before we departed, she hugged me again. Truly, how blessed I felt to be loved in that passing moment by such a loving and lively spirit.

From that day forward, whenever Emma and I saw each other, we hugged and said to one another, "I love you. You are so wonderful!" This usual greeting never stopped uplifting me and always stirred within me an all-encompassing sense of peace and love. What a wonderful way to greet another human being! What a wonderful thing to do each day!

What if we all could love like that, I began to think, *if we all could reach out to one another, stranger, enemy, and friend alike and say, I love you, you are wonderful, so wonderful, and really see the wonder and mystery within the other's eyes.* If only, like Emma, we could suspend judgment, even if for only a few short moments, and see beyond those all too human flaws and imperfections that we all have and see the light, love, and beauty within and know that every human too has suffered, just like we have.

Wow! How glorious it would be to be able to get past the ego, with its distorted judgments and labels that prevent us from knowing and loving other people fully. Maybe someday in the distant future we will all be able to love like Emma, and to hug one another and say, "I love you. You are wonderful, so wonderful!" It is a difficult task, yet I to think that someday it can happen.

42

HEALING THE BROKENNESS WITHIN

Essential points

- ◆ Look for the emotion behind the words.
- ◆ Aspire to heal the brokenness within yourself and the world.

A young woman once told me about her grandfather, who was a resident at an Alzheimer's care unit. She remembered him as sweet and kind, but he now had moments when he flared in anger and yelled at the top of his lungs, "I want my little red wagon back! You took my little red wagon and I want it back now!" Whoever happened to be there at the time received the brunt of his anger, usually with clenched fists, a seizing of the collar or a good box in the ears. One day he slugged another resident, while repeating those words.

It was most unusual, the young woman thought, because she had never seen her grandfather behave like that, yet she knew that he once had a little red wagon. She told me how he came from a poor immigrant family. When he was a child, he never had many toys, but he wanted more than anything else a beautiful shiny red wagon that he saw one day in a store window. When his parents saw that, they saved enough money to buy it and surprised him. How happy he was with his new toy, but not long afterwards when he was outside playing, the boy next door took his brand new shiny red wagon and did not want to return it.

I reflected on that story because I have come to realize that so many of the elders I have worked with have reoccurring memories of some poignant incident from childhood or adolescence. I could not help reflecting on our own inner tapes that keep playing the same story, the same wound, often manifested in a different guise. It is as if they come back to be heard and healed.

When I was five years old I was playing on the street with a group of older children. They were playing ball, and I was too young to play in their quick, rough, and agile way, yet I wanted to have someone to play with. What I really wanted more than anything was attention. I wanted to be heard, so I picked up a sharp broken piece of glass from a shattered coke bottle and squeezed a piece into my thumb until it started to bleed.

I remember crying because it hurt, yet really I was crying about something else. There was another wound behind that one: my father's death the year before. Everything was hushed in the house. No one wanted to talk about death. No one explained what it really meant: my father was not coming back. Instead, I kept waiting with a sad and heavy heart. Unable to express the pain I felt inside, this was the opportunity for me to express it through the broken glass and to say *listen, someone, anyone, I am hurting.*

When that young woman mentioned the red wagon, it reminded me of how important it is to take the broken pieces within ourselves and to make them whole again. In the Jewish tradition, there is this idea that the world is like a broken vessel, and it is up to each one of us to take the shattered pieces and help make them whole again. By healing the brokenness within ourselves, we are healing the brokenness within the world and are helping to make the vessel whole. And by helping to heal others, we are also helping to heal ourselves.

My work has been about helping to facilitate the healing of the brokenness in the elders I have served, not as a priest or psychotherapist, or what some people would call "healer," but in my own way, be it as a massage therapist, activity therapist, elder care advocate or social service worker. My hope is that I have in some way made their journey a little lighter, freer, and more whole. Yet without my intending it, through their healing, I have helped facilitate my own. That exchange and interchange has always been magical, alchemical, and sacred to me. I have come to realize how important it is to mend the brokenness within ourselves and within the world. It is our responsibility.

Suggestions for creating meaningful and engaged activities

Creating "wish" or "worry dolls" is a wonderful way for elders to create new friendships and build community. This activity can easily be adapted for groups or individuals.

♦ Gather materials such as popsicle sticks, tongue depressors, or old fashioned clothes pins, colored pipe cleaners cut in half, small squares of colorful fabric, small strips of colored paper, clay or Model Magic, pens and scissors, glue sticks, feathers, glitter, ribbons, sequins, buttons, bows, little Styrofoam balls or shapes that can be used for a head, googly eyes and anything else that can be glued onto the doll.

♦ Ask each elder to choose one popsicle stick (or tongue depressor or clothes pin), one strip of paper to write down a wish or worry, one fabric, and one pipe cleaner.

♦ Ask your elders to think about their wishes, their hopes, or their worries, grief, or any distressing thoughts which play over and over again in their minds. If they feel comfortable sharing, ask them to share.

- ◆ Ask them to write down the wish or worry on the little scrap of paper.
  - Then wrap the paper around the popsicle stick or clothes pin.
  - Wrap the fabric around the paper.
  - Take the pipe cleaners and wrap them tightly around the fabric, leaving the ends out.
  - Make the doll with the other fun stuff!
  - Give the doll a name.
  - Ask the doll what she needs from you and/or what the solution is.

The elders can then put their dolls in a special place where they can easily be picked up when the wish or worry comes, and ask the doll for guidance as to what they can do to bring resolution.

CHAPTER

43

THE POWER OF LOVE

Essential points

- ♦ Aspire to be a channel for love.
- ♦ Stay on purpose.
- ♦ Do what is meaningful for you and for others, and joy will follow.
- ♦ Bring joy to those who need it most, and bliss will follow.

We are all just passing through.

Turning the calendar, day by day, week by week, month by month, year by year, I ask, *Already, that quickly? Where did the time go?*

Each year, time seems to move more swiftly. Sometimes I want to make time stop or slow it down for just one minute to catch up with all the things I want to do, yet I always have to ask, *Am I doing what is most important? Am I doing what is most meaningful and essential? Am I living my life in rhythm to the larger pulse?*

For people like Helen, time moves in a vastly different way. Most of her days are spent in bed. Forgetting time and how much time has passed, she marks Xs with black marker each day on a calendar on the wall by the side of her bed. Often she looks at the marks, forgetful of whether her latest X was placed today or yesterday. With each passing month, her calendar became filled with nothing but Xs in black marker. Each day she asked what day it was, and "Is it marked on the calendar?" If not, she asked me to mark it for her.

Helen didn't have many visitors. At 104, she had outlived her daughter, son and their children, who had no children.

Often I am asked, "Isn't the kind of work you do depressing? To be around all those sick and dying people?" The truth is we are all dying. From the moment we are born we begin to die, and like the elders I have worked with, we are all just visitors passing through, be it through skilled nursing or life. It gives me infinite joy knowing that I have in some small way touched someone's heart, that I have made a difference in someone's life by making it just a little bit better.

Helen once told me that my daily visits were what she looked forward to most of all in the day, adding a bright spot in her life. With one day bleeding into the next, she rarely turned the TV on, except to watch the news. Much of the time she slept. Within a moment of my arrival, she would open her eyes and exclaim, "How happy I am to see you, dear." A smile would suddenly appear on her face as she lifted her arms, then clasped her hands together, pressing them to her heart. Bending down to kiss her, I would give her a hug.

Helen's body was thin and frail. I could feel more bones than flesh. Putting my hand in hers, I would sit next to her. Her face seemed to glow and come alive again, as we simply looked at one another for a few moments.

There were no words, yet it was as if a bigger life force was at play. I call it love, and such moments make the work I do joyful and vital, not sad. During those times I can say, *yes, I am doing the essential, the most important. I am doing what is mean-ingful for me.*

Helen often put her hand to her heart and said, "How I wish I had a piece of candy to give to you today. It would make me so happy if I could offer you one." One day she excitedly asked me to open the drawer of her night table. Inside was a box of See's. "Have a piece of candy, honey," she said with enthusiasm.

How could I refuse? She watched while I chewed the luscious piece of chocolate, with caramel melting on my tongue. "It's delicious," I said, letting the flavor linger.

Helen clasped her hands together in a gesture of *I am so happy that you like it.* This simple act of offering a piece of candy to someone you care about meant a lot to Helen. How happy she was. And how happy I was to see the joy on her face and to taste the candy.

"Have another, dear." she said. I had another, then closed the box and put it away.

Twice a month, Helen's caregiver helped her put on a pair of slacks with a pullover and assisted her in her wheelchair to the beauty parlor to have her hair done and apply rouge and lipstick. Afterwards, she would excitedly ask her caregiver to find me.

"You look beautiful," I exclaimed, kissing her on the cheeks, then standing back to look into her eyes that sparkled with renewed life and joy.

Helen liked asking questions. Although I had asked her often about her life, rarely did she talk about it. She always turned the conversation around to questions like: *What was your day like? What is your family like? Oh my, you mean they all passed on already? Are you married? No, well I will pray that you meet a good man.*

Although she had a hard time keeping track of the days, she had a surprisingly good memory at age 104. She never asked the same question more than once. She enjoyed hearing about my life and remembered all the details of my life.

I have found that one of the best antidotes for any kind of sadness or loneliness is to step out of yourself and listen to another.

Each day that I saw Helen, she told me of her prayers, "How I want the best for you. I pray that you are happy, that you are protected by angels, that your life is good, and most important, that you are not alone anymore. I pray that you will meet a good man to marry. When I go to sleep at night, I see your face and this is what I pray. When I wake up in the morning I see your face again, and I say another prayer for you."

How touched I was by her kind gesture. I knew she meant every word. Her good wishes and prayers will be with me always. I still feel their blessings even now while I write these words, as I wonder, looking over at my husband reading by the window overlooking the hills with pine trees shrouded in mist: *Did her prayers help bring him to me, a good man, just like she prayed, one whom I adore, who brings me much joy and happiness?*

I cannot answer that question. I do not know, but what I do know is this: it is all about love, love, love… There is only love. Through love all things can heal, can grow, can mend and transform and make one's heart sing with elation. The elders I have served have touched and changed me as much as I have them, all through the spirit of love. Love is magical, the most powerful tool there is that can restore all things, and even make people who were about to die, live…

ON WORKING WITH
PEOPLE LIVING WITH ALZHEIMER'S

(See chapters 6, 8, 9, 10, 11, 14, 15, 16, 23, 25, 31, 32,
33, 36, 38, 39, 40, 41, 42)

a. Personal reflections

♦ The creative arts are a wonderful way to connect with people living with Alzheimer's.

♦ If you happen to live in New York or on the East Coast, I highly recommend visiting the Museum of Modern Art. They have a special program for people with Alzheimer's disease called *Meet Me at MoMA*. They also published two marvelous books that contain a DVD illustrating how the program works. Please see suggested reading section for titles and website address.

♦ Inspired by MoMA's program, the Frye Museum in Seattle, Washington, has a similar program offering workshops for family caregivers and professionals. I've taken one of their workshops and highly recommend it.

- *I'm Still Here*, by Dr. John Zeisel, a champion of using the creative arts to connect with people challenged by Alzheimer's, is another book I highly recommend. Please see my reading and resource list for other suggestions.

- Windows, nature, and sunlight are all extremely important for individuals who have Alzheimer's. Windows with a view enable them to witness the changing of days and seasons. Plant colorful flowers outside, and have a bird aviary or butterfly garden.

b. Suggestions for creating engaging and inspiring activities

- Any of the suggested activities throughout this book can be modified for working with people who have Alzheimer's. Of special interest in the creative arts please see end notes of chapters 4, 5, and 23. Of special interest in the therapeutic benefits of nature please see end notes of chapter 22.

- **Painting in watercolors.** Although there are many ways to experiment with watercolors, I am most familiar with the following:

  - Invite your elders to choose their favorite image or images from magazines or books—flowers, trees, landscapes, etc., and to paint the images with watercolors! Remind them to not worry about the end result. It doesn't even have to look like the original picture! All they need to do is simply paint, have fun, and enjoy the process.

  - Invite your elders to paint free style. After wetting the paper with a sponge, dip brush into paint, and let the paint drop from the brush onto the paper. Try using different colors, allowing them to run into each other. Play with the color and have fun! They can also draw shapes with only water on the brush, then drop paint onto the watery shapes. Try experimenting using salt.

It will draw the color towards it, as well as add a grainy texture to the painting.

- Be sure to use high quality paper, ninety pound paper or above. You might also want to use watercolor pencils and crayons, both of which dissolve in water and are easy to use. If water colors don't seem right, try tempera markers, glitter markers, or water color pencils or crayons on their own. There are some stunning utensils available at any arts and crafts store. I have even found some nice ones at Target.

♦ **Group painting.** This works well if you have an art teacher facilitating, or if you happen to be skilled at painting or drawing. This activity gives everyone the opportunity to participate, even those who might not be able to hold a brush in their hand. Invite the group to choose a setting. For example, a forest path, the ocean, animals in a garden, etc. Whatever they choose, invite them to be imaginative and create as a group. Each elder has the opportunity to contribute what he or she would like to see in the picture, e.g., "put a bridge there," "a yellow leaf here," "a flower there," or "how about a stone or big rock here?" Encourage them to be as bold and imaginative as they like. There are no wrong or right ways, and a group endeavor is especially nice.

♦ **Music.** This activity works with almost everyone, and especially for elders who might be in more advanced stages of Alzheimer's. Discover their favorite songs and record or download them onto an iPod or any other listening device with headphones and play. For an example of the uplifting impact on an elder, please see this touching video on YouTube called, *Old Man in Nursing Home Reacting to Hearing Music from His Era.*

Some questions to think about:

- What did they grow up listening to?

- What was their wedding song?

- What music was associated with some of the highest points in their lives, like falling in love with their spouse?

- What is their favorite kind of music? Classical, Jazz, rock and roll, folk, pop, world music like African, Indian, or Middle Eastern?

- Do certain rhythms and songs perk them up and make them want to move or dance?

♦ **Memory joggers.** Surround each elder with things with which he or she is familiar, such as old quilts, wall hangings, old furniture, old dolls, teddy bears, books, and photographs anything that is a part of his or her past. Create a memory box with old photos and other items that hold precious memories.

♦ **Trivia. (see chapter 33)**

♦ **Start a massage therapy program at your residential care community.** Arrange for a massage therapist to work with your elders for one or two hours once or twice a month, or more if your budget allows. He or she can work with your elders doing one-on-one room visits or as a group activity, each individual receiving a 10-15 minute massage, with essential oils and music creating a peaceful ambience for healing. Massage can work wonders, helping with anxiety, restlessness, stiff muscles and joints. It can also help an elder feel more connected in the world and to others. When someone is no longer able communicate through words, touch can work wonders. **(also see chapters 11, 13, 14)**

♦ **Playing with dolls and stuffed animals**. Don't shy away from these items, judging them as childish. They can bring a sense of security and give someone the opportunity to love again. To love the baby she once had. To show affection to the animal he may no longer have. Love is miraculously healing! (**see chapter 32**)

♦ **Sensory stimulation box or cart**. Some objects I like to use are:

- Those that appeal to the **sense of smell**, such as essential oils like rose, lavender, or orange blossom; spices such as cinnamon, cloves and vanilla; and chocolate or coffee.

- Those that appeal to the **sense of hearing**, such as the sound of bells (I have also used Tibetan singing bells and bowls), recorded sounds of a didgeridoo; flutes; chimes; ocean waves; running streams in a forest; birds chirping; whales or dolphins; the breaking of a potato chip.

- Those that appeal to the **sense of taste** such as the saltiness of a saltine or potato chip; something sweet like chocolate, a raisin, or apple sauce; something tart like an orange (modified according to an elder who may have allergies, be diabetic or on a pureed diet).

- Those that **appeal to touch** like a piece of velvet, faux fur, silk, sand, shells, sand paper, a ball of yarn, and/or smooth glossy round rocks. (**see chapter 16**).

- Those that **appeal to sight** such as colorful pictures of flowers (or a real flower which invites touch); birds; trees; animals; natural settings such as a forest; a river; a meadow; or an ocean; paintings; or places around the world.

c. The difference between dementia and Alzheimer's:

♦ *Dementia* is an umbrella term used for loss of memory and other mental impairments severe enough to interfere with daily life, caused by physical changes in the brain. Some of the more common types of dementia are Alzheimer's disease, vascular dementia, dementia with Lewy bodies, frontotemporal dementia, and Parkinson's. For more specific detailed information on the characteristics of each one, please see http://www.alz.org/dementia/types-of-dementia.asp.

d. Tips on communicating with someone who has Alzheimer's (Please see Alzheimer's Association at www.alz.org):

♦ **Be patient and supportive.** Let the person know you're listening and trying to understand. Show the person that you care about what she is saying and be careful not to interrupt.

♦ **Offer comfort and reassurance.** If the person is having trouble communicating, let him know that it's okay. Encourage the person to continue to explain his thoughts.

♦ **Avoid criticizing or correcting.** Don't tell the person what she is saying is incorrect. Instead, listen and try to find the meaning in what is being said. Repeat what was said if it helps to clarify the thought.

♦ **Avoid arguing.** If the person says something you don't agree with, let it be. Arguing usually only makes things worse — often heightening the level of agitation for the person with dementia.

♦ **Offer a guess.** If the person uses the wrong word or cannot find a word, try guessing the right one. If you understand what the person means, you may not need to give the correct word. Be careful not to cause unnecessary frustration.

♦ **Encourage unspoken communication.** If you don't understand what is being said, ask the person to point or gesture.

♦ **Limit distractions.** Find a place that's quiet. The surroundings should support the person's ability to focus on his thoughts.

♦ **Focus on feelings, not facts.** Sometimes the emotions being expressed are more important than what is being said. Look for the feelings behind the words. Tone of voice and other actions may provide clues.

While a person with later-stage Alzheimer's may not always respond, he or she still benefits from continued communication and your presence. When words fail, touch can be a powerful tool for connecting. For some people touch might be inappropriate and even stir up anxiety, but for many it can be reassuring and calming. When communicating, it's important to choose your words carefully.

♦ **Identify yourself.** Approach the person from the front and say who you are. Make eye contact; if the person is seated or reclined, go down to that level.

♦ **Call the person by name.** This helps orient the person and gets her attention. Ongoing communication is important, no matter how difficult it may become or how confused the person with Alzheimer's or dementia may appear.

♦ **Use short, simple words and sentences.** Lengthy requests or stories can be overwhelming. Ask one question at a time. Give one-step directions.

♦ **Speak slowly and distinctively.** Be aware of speed and clarity. Use a gentle and relaxed tone — a lower pitch is more calming.

♦ **Patiently wait for a response.** The person may need extra time to process what you said.

♦ **Repeat information or questions as needed.** If the person doesn't respond, wait a moment. Then ask again.

♦ **Repeat what you don't understand.**

♦ **Match the person's emotional tone when repeating what he or she said.**

♦ **Validate the feeling the person expresses.**

♦ **Use touch to confirm feeling, but only if the person is open to it.**

♦ **Avoid confusing and vague statements.** If you tell the person to "Hop in!" she may interpret your instructions literally. Instead, describe the action directly: "Please come here. Your shower is ready." Instead of using "it" or "that," name the object or place. For example, rather than, "Here it is," say "Here is your hat."

♦ **Turn negatives into positives.** Instead of saying, "Don't go there," say, "Let's go here."

♦ **Give visual cues.** To help demonstrate the task, point or touch the item you want the individual to use or begin the task for the person.

♦ **Avoid quizzing.** Reminiscing may be healthy, but avoid asking, "Do you remember when … ?"

♦ **Write things down.** Try using written notes as reminders if the person is able to understand them.

♦ **Treat the person with dignity and respect.** Avoid talking down to the person or talking as if he isn't there. Talk directly to the person. Avoid talking to as if he were a child.

♦ **Convey an easygoing manner.** Be aware of your feelings and attitude — you may be communicating through your tone of voice. Use positive, friendly facial expressions and nonverbal communication.

e. **The following suggestions include and build on those presented in John Zeisel's book *I'm Still Here* (p.185-187):**

◆ **Create a living space that in not confusing.** Place items that the person uses in an area easy to find. If he likes sitting in a particular chair, be sure the path getting there is clear and free from any confusion or clutter.

I find that labeling cabinets or drawers in clear block letters makes it easy to navigate.

(Labelers are great!) If he likes to use a particular drinking glass or cup, label those items outside the cabinet. You can label just about any item that he uses often and will appreciate having the reminder.

◆ **Plan what you will talk about.** Don't expect a conversation to arise on its own. Take the lead. Share how your day went, what you did, what you know about his day, as well as what you do in your job. Discuss any subject you think she might enjoy. Bring a magazine article or newspaper clipping that she might enjoy discussing. If she liked travel, talk about travel. If it is architecture or art, talk about that. If you are a family caregiver, share moments from your life together, his job, or your family. Whatever it is, prepare what you will talk about.

I always prepare but also believe it is important to not be too attached to the plan. Look for what inspires her as you are discussing a topic. If you notice sparks of inspiration, use that as an opportunity to ask more questions. Sometimes those questions open other discussions, which you did not plan, but are relevant to her life. Use those sparks to direct your conversation and let go of your plan.

I had a client who had a life-long interest in birds, so I brought a book with pictures of birds for us to discuss. As we were looking, he said, "I wonder why so many varieties of birds were created." "A great question," I replied. He said, "I think we should ask god." The subject of birds opened up an unplanned conversation about god, religion, and his childhood as an altar boy.

◆ **Surround the person with familiar items.** Keep favorite photos, wall hangings, paintings, pieces of furniture, and any other objects or memorabilia around him. Use these objects as points of conversation. If he had a favorite shirt or cap, be sure he has it and can wear it when he wants. If he had a favorite quilt or blanket, keep that on his bed.

◆ **Bring images that can be used to communicate.** Share newspaper clippings from what happened in the world on the day she was born, or on other days that were significant to her. Bring family photos, wedding videos, or any family videos or pictures. What about any awards? Or photos of places that she may have a special connection to. What about special objects from a trip that she took or a special gift that she treasured?

I also find that almost everyone is touched by an uplifting animal story. Often I bring animal magazines with heartwarming stories and pictures to share. This always evokes a smile.

◆ **Create a record of your visits.** Decide what kind of record you will leave. You can use a wall calendar or visitor's book that you write in each time you visit.

What can be a fun creative project is to design your own visitor's book together, using his favorite colored paper or fabric, favorite images or photos, anything that might hold a special meaning for him. Be as creative as you like. Inside you can record your visit along with what you did, anything of special importance about the visit, or any visuals such as a newspaper or magazine clipping that he especially liked.

LESSONS I HAVE GATHERED FROM THIS JOURNEY

1. **It is easy to forget about the *gifts* that come from illness, loss, or hardship, but I have learned that gifts come with all things.** If you love someone who has dementia, learn to see the gifts, and if possible, accept those gifts with grace, love, and gratitude. I have learned from people who have dementia:

   - To slow down and be more patient.

   - To be more present. If I am not present, I will not be able to fully see or understand the other person.

   - To leave my world behind, along with my definition of reality.

   - To meet the person where he or she is now, without any expectations or judgments.

   - To listen, although I may not understand.

   - To love unconditionally. The human spirit always recognizes love and responds to love.

   - To surrender to what is. If something cannot be changed,

work with it instead of against it. By working against it, you make it harder for yourself and the other person.

♦ To see beyond the surface. Look for the light within. It is still there but it just might take a little digging and more SEEING.

♦ I worked with one elder who made me pause when I realized how thankful I was to her. My day had been hectic. I was trying to *fit too many things into one day,* and in the midst of being with her, I suddenly realized how she was there to teach me. I reached for her hand, looked into her eyes, told her about my day, and said, "Thank you. You've taught me so much about the importance of being patient, slowing down, and being present. I will always be thankful to you." She looked at me, completely present and alert, her eyes twinkling with love, and smiled. Then she spoke very clearly, "Really? I'm so glad." It was a precious moment I will always remember with love and gratitude.

2. The best gift you can give anyone is being PRESENT.

♦ Your time and presence are infinitely more important than anything else. Listen wholeheartedly. Be there with the person, not somewhere else. BE HERE NOW, FULLY PRESENT.

♦ Don't run away or avoid your loved one out of fear or discomfort. If you are a family caregiver who struggles with this, work with a trained professional, such as a care manager or psychotherapist, who will be able to help you get through your difficulties.

3. Don't take anger personally!

♦ Learn what is beneath the anger that needs to be addressed.

Sometimes it appears as if the anger is about one thing, but the deeper you dig, the more you discover it is about something else, and something else beneath that. (**see chapter 34**)

♦ Stay centered as best as you can and remind yourself that you might be angry, too if you suddenly had to move to an unfamiliar environment surrounded by a lot of strangers and could no longer do what you once enjoyed. Imagine if every time you had to go to the bathroom, you had to call for a caregiver to help you, and you might have to wait longer than you'd like because others need assistance too, and the care community is understaffed! Be patient and understanding. Your role as son or daughter is changing, and so is your loved one's role as a parent.

♦ If your anger goes beyond the current situation, and is an issue you've had to deal with earlier in your life together, consider working with a psychotherapist if your parent is open to it.

4. **Never say goodbye to anyone when you are angry.** If you are angry, pause, take a breath, center yourself, and remember life is short. We never know when it may be our last breath, or theirs. If it is your time or theirs, it is better to know that we said goodbye with love.

5. **Learn to let go and forgive. Forgiveness is miraculously healing!**

♦ Let go of anger, resentment, and bitterness. It will lighten your load and bring more peace and love into your heart. If you are holding a grudge against or are angry with anyone in your life, try to open a healing conversation with that person. If that is not possible, write a letter to the person, and remember that he or she, too is human, and has also suffered.

♦ When I leave this planet, I want to leave light and free.

6. **"If not now, when?"** This quote from Hillel is something we should all live by.

 ♦ When I forget, I later regret! So often we put things off to future—the future that may never come. If something is truly important, do it now, don't keep it on the list of things to do some day.

7. **If you or your loved one have not done an Advanced Directive, get one done.**

 ♦ Ask your doctor for one, or you can find the form on line by going to the website www.caringinfo.org

 ♦ If an Advanced Directive feels too overwhelming, as it is for many, have a heart-to-heart discussion with your loved ones about your wishes.

 ♦ Or simply write a letter to your doctor stating your wishes. Please see The Letter Project at Stanford at http://med. stanford.edu/letter. This highly commendable project makes your wishes known through a very simple, short, user-friendly, and enjoyable form. The letter is available in several languages including Hindi, Tagalog, Mandarin, Urdu, Farsi, Spanish, German, and Russian.

 ♦ Talking about death is not easy for anyone, but it is important to discuss any last wishes, requests, and funeral arrangements. For a lighter, more entertaining way of opening up a discussion, use a deck of cards called the *Go Wish Game, Decide What's Important Together.* You can purchase them on line for under $10 at codaalliance.org.

 ♦ My mother was one of the most conscientious and thoughtful people I know when it came to her own death, and she taught me a lot about preparing for death. Years before she passed away, when she was still young and vibrant, she showed me where all her important papers were kept. On the shelf next to those papers, she had a cardboard shoe box where she kept a simple but pretty sky blue chiffon dress, a pair of shoes, stockings, rosary beads, and her old prayer book. Warning me that the funeral director would try to sell me expensive clothing, accessories, and casket, she admonished me in her sweet, soft-spoken wise way, "Be careful, Mary Ann. Don't let them sell you all kinds of expensive things. Don't let them make you feel guilty. I don't need an expensive box. All I ask for is something white, simple, and sturdy. Everything I want to be buried in is right here in this box." She also had purchased her own plot next to my father and the rest of the family, and she showed me the receipt, the contract, and the map with the location of the plot. Knowing I was the last family member left, my mother did not want to make it difficult for me by leaving a mess to sort through and clean. Photo albums, family heirlooms, handmade crocheted blankets, and anything else she knew I wanted to keep, she organized and put into labeled boxes.

In her approach to death and dying, she was my teacher. I will always be thankful.

8. **Allow your loved one to help you, if he or she wishes.** Helping gives us a sense of purpose, no matter how small the task may be.

   ♦ Recently, one resident sitting in her wheelchair at a care center, kept tapping me on the rump. I repeatedly asked what she wanted but couldn't understand until finally she gestured that my belt tie was undone, and she wanted to tie it. As her arthritic shaky fingers fumbled against my rump, I exercised patience for what seemed an interminably long time. When she finally finished, she looked so pleased!

9. **Learn to surrender to the process of living, aging, and dying. Have the courage and wisdom to recognize when to let go.**

   ♦ Do all you can to prolong your life and stay healthy and vital, but sooner or later, accept that the body changes whether we want it to or not. In Atul Gawande's book, *Being Mortal*, he vividly describes the process that occurs in the aging body (pp. 29-31). It cannot be prevented. It simply happens.

   ♦ We live in a dysfunctional society that denies death and turns aging into a disgrace, an abnormality. Nader Robert Shabahangi, founder of AgeSong, wrote a book entitled *Faces of Aging* to accompany his stunning collection of photographs of elders. The faces he captures shine with light, wisdom, and an exquisite beauty in all their wrinkles. We need more faces like that on the covers of magazines — new role models for a changed society of how we view aging.

   ♦ Behind all the fighting to keep our youth through plastic surgery or other means, there seems to be an emptiness, a denial of life as it is, in all its wondrous changes. Growing old is not always pleasant or easy, but with everything in life there is something of great value that comes — gifts waiting to be received. Part of surrendering to the process is being able to recognize those gifts.

   ♦ Life is impermanent. So is youth. If the quality of my life were to become severely compromised, I don't want to prolong it through artificial means or expensive treatments. I want to age naturally, with grace and dignity. I hope to die that way too.

10. **Remember to stop, breathe, and take care of yourself.** Often we, as caregivers, forget to take care of our own needs.

It is essential that we do so. Remember that if you aren't taken care of, you can't take care of anyone else. Get a massage, take a walk, read your favorite book, sign up for a class that looks exciting, go on a weekend getaway!

11. **Be grateful for life. It is a gift.** Each moment, each breath is an act of grace, a blessing to be used wisely. Remember to be grateful for the good and not so good, alike, because no matter how difficult or challenging life can be, there is always a lesson to be gained.

APPENDIX III

SUGGESTED READING AND RESOURCES

Basting, Anne Davis. *Forget Memory: Creating Better Lives for People With Dementia*. Baltimore: John Hopkins University Press, 2009.

Brackey, Jolene. *Creating Moments of Joy for the Person with Alzheimer's or Dementia: A Journal for Caregivers*. Purdue: Purdue University Press, 2008.

Callanan, Maggie, and Patricia Kelly. *Final Gifts: Understanding the Special Awareness, Needs, and Communications of the Dying*. New York: Simon and Schuster, 2012.

Coste, Joanne Koenig. *Learning to Speak Alzheimer's*. Boston: Houghton Mifflin Company, 2003.

Darley, Suzanne, and Wende Heath. *The Expressive Arts Activity Book: A Resource for Professionals*. London: Jessica Kingsley Publishers, 2008.

Das, Ram. *Still Here: Embracing Aging, Changing, and Dying*. New York: Riverhead Books, 2001.

Frankl, Viktor. *Man's Search for Meaning*. New York: Beacon Press, 2006.

Gawande, Atul. *Being mortal*. New York: Metropolitan Books, Henry Holt and Company, 2014.

Killick, John, and Claire Craig. *Creativity and Communication in Persons with Dementia: A Practical Guide.* London: Jessica Kingsley Publishers, 2012.

Konnikova, Maria. *The Power of Touch, The New Yorker,* March 5, 2015.

Matzkin, Alice, and Richard Matzkin. *The Art of Aging: Celebrating the Authentic Aging Self.* Boulder: Sentient Publications, 2009.

The Museum of Modern Art. *Meetme: Making Art Accessible to People with Dementia.* New York: The Museum of Modern Art, 2009.

The Museum of Modern Art. *Meetme Art Modules: Making Art Accessible to People with Dementia.* New York: The Museum of Modern Art, 2009.

Ornish, Dean. *Love and Survival: 8 Pathways to Intimacy and Health.* New York: Harper Collins, 1999.

Rehmen, Naomi, Rachel. *Kitchen Table Wisdom: Stories that Heal.* New York: Riverhead Books, 2006.

Rehmen, Naomi, Rachel. *My Grandfather's Blessings: Stories of Strength, Refuge, and Belonging.* New York: Riverhead Books, 2001.

Sacks, Oliver. *Gratitude.* New York: Alfred A. Knopf, 2015.

Schachter-Shalomi, Zalman, and Ronald S. Miller. *From Age-Ing to Sage-Ing: A Revolutionary Approach to Growing Older.* New York: Time Warner Books, 2014.

Shabahangi, Nader Robert. *Faces of Aging.* Warsaw: Elders Academy Press, 2002.

Shouse, Deborah. *Connecting in the Land of Dementia.* Las Vegas: Central Recovery Press, 2016.

Thomas, Bill. *Second Wind: Navigating the Passage to a Slower, Deeper, and More Connected Life.* New York: Simon and Schuster, 2015.

Whitehouse, J. Peter. *The Myth of Alzheimer's: What You Aren't Being Told About Today's Most Dreaded Diagnosis.* New York: St. Martin's Griffin, 2008.

Zeisel, John. *I'm Still Here: A New Philosophy of Alzheimer's Care.* New York: Avery, Penguin Group, 2010.

ADULT COLORING BOOKS FOR PEACE AND RELAXATION

Agredo, Mary, and Javier Agredo. *Creative Haven Hamsa Designs Coloring Book.* New York: Dover Publications, 2014.

Media, Adam. *Stress-less Coloring: Flower Patterns: 100+ Coloring Pages for Peace and Relaxation.* Avon, MA: Adams Media, 2015.

Gogarty, Jim. *The Mandala Coloring Book: Inspire Creativity, Reduce Stress, and Bring Balance with 100 Coloring Pages.* Avon, MA: Adams Media, 2013.

Levin, Freddie and Judy Dick. *Shalom Coloring: Adult Coloring Book.* Springfield, N.J.: Behrman, 2015.

POETRY

Behn, Robin, and Chase Twichell. *The Practice of Poetry: Writing Exercises from Poets Who Teach.* New York: Harper Perennial, 1992.

Cummings, E.E. *Selected Poems.* New York: Liveright, 2007.

Hass, Robert, and Stephen Mitchell. *Into the Garden: A Wedding Anthology.* New York: HarperCollins, 1993.

Housden, Roger. *Ten Poems to Open Your Heart.* New York: Harmony Books, 2002.

Gibran, Kahlil. *The Prophet.* New York: Alfred A. Knopf, 1979.

Hafiz, and translator Daniel Ladinsky. *The Subject Tonight Is Love: 60 Wild and Sweet Poems of Hafiz.* Myrtle Beach, South Carolina: Pumpkin House Press, 1996.

Joseph, Jenny. *When I Grow Old I Shall Wear Purple.* London: Souvenir Press, 2001.

Ladinsky, Daniel. *I Heard God Laughing: Renderings of Hafiz.* Walnut Creek, CA: Sufism Reoriented, 1996.

McDowell, Robert. *Poetry as Spiritual Practice: Reading, Writing, and Using Poetry in your Daily Rituals, Aspirations, and Intentions.* New York: Free Press, 2008.

Mitchell, Stephen. *The Enlightened Heart: An Anthology of Sacred Poetry.* New York: Harper Perennial, 1993.

Mosley, Ivo. *Earth Poems.* New York: Harper San Francisco, 1996.

Oliver, Mary. *The Leaf and the Cloud.* Boston: De Capo Press, 2000.

Oliver, Mary. *New and Selected Poems.* Boston: Beacon Press, 1992.

Oliver, Mary. *Why I Wake Early.* Boston: Beacon Press, 2005.

Rumi, Jalal al-Din, translation by Coleman Barks and John Moyne. *The Essential Rumi.* San Francisco: Harper One, 2004.

Tagore, Rabindranath. *Gitanjali.*

Williams, Oscar, and Edwin Honig. *The Mentor Book of Major American Poets.* New York: Mentor Books, 1962.

Roberts, Elizabeth, and Elias Amidon. *Life Prayers from Around the World.* New York: Harper San Francisco, 1996.

Creating a Living Legacy

Birren, James, and Kathyrn N. Cochran. *Telling the Stories of Life Through Guided Autobiography Groups.* Baltimore, Maryland: John Hopkins University Press, 2001.

Campbell, Richard, and Cheryl Svensson. *Writing Your Legacy: The Step-by-Step Guide to Crafting Your Life Story.* Blue Ash, Ohio: Writer's Digest, 2015.

Franco, Carol, and Kent Lineback. *The Legacy Guide: Capturing the Facts, Memories, and Meaning of Your Life.* New York: Jeremy P. Tarcher/Penguin, 2006.

Polce-Lynch, Mary. *Nothing Left Unsaid: Creating a Healing Legacy with Final Letter, Words, and Letters.* New York: Marlowe and Company, 2006.

Spence, Linda. *Legacy: A Step-by-Step Guide to Writing Personal History.* Athens, Ohio: Swallow Press/Ohio University Press, 1997.

Recommended films and documentaries

Being Mortal
Old man in nursing home reacting to hearing music from his era
(You tube video)
The Alzheimer's Project
Complaints of A Dutiful Daughter
I Remember when I Paint
First Cousin Once Removed
Dementia with Dignity
Alive Inside
Iris
Caregiver Wellness

Creative Arts Organizations for Elders

www.moma.org/meetmet/: An art program designed by The Museum of Modern Art (MoMA) for people living with dementia.

www.eldergivers.org: Art with Elders (AWE) offers programs to older adults living in long-term care facilities in the San Francisco Bay Area, providing the opportunity to explore and develop latent artistic talents. Art with Elders' mission is to connect the generations by celebrating the wisdom, talents, and creativity of older adults.

www.estanyc.org: Elders Share the Arts is a Brooklyn based organization offering a wide variety of creative arts programming that ignites creative expression, cultivates elders' role as bearers of history and culture, and generates new pathways to connect them to their communities. They also offer training programs for organizations interested in creative aging.

www.aftaarts.org: Arts for the Aging (AFTA) is based in the greater Washington D.C. area. This nonprofit outreach organization brings a wide variety of creative arts programs, which include visual, literary, musical, performing, multidisciplinary, and intergenerational offerings to elders in care centers, skilled nursing, assisted living, and community centers.

www.fryemueseum.org/program/here-now: a Seattle based museum that offers an art program similar to MoMA's Meet Me. Designed for elders with dementia, *here:now* is six week program that includes gallery tours and art making in the studio. The museum also offers workshops to caregivers and professionals working with elders.

https://www.scrippsoma.org: Opening Minds through Art (OMA) is an intergenerational art program for people with dementia. It is grounded in person-centered ethics and founded on the fact that people with dementia are capable of expressing themselves creatively.

Other Organizations of Interest
www.ahcancal.org: American Health Care Association, whose membership includes long-term care and post-acute care providers, advocates for quality care and services for frail, elderly, and disabled Americans.

www.Alzfdn.org: Alzheimer's Foundation of America (AFA) provides services for helping people with dementia and their families.

www.alz.org: Alzheimer's Association provides services for helping people with dementia and their families.

www.caringinfo.org: Caring Info is a program of the National Hospice and Palliative Care Organization providing free resources to help people make decisions about end-of-life care and services before a crisis.

www.codaalliance.org: A collaboration of individuals and representatives in the San Jose/Silicon Valley, California area from local hospices, hospitals, faith communities, universities, and elder care organizations dedicated to the mission of implementing social change in end-of-life-care.

www.edenalt.org: The Eden Alternative is a non-profit organization dedicated to improving the well-being of elders and their care partners by transforming the communities in which they live and work.

www.eldercare.gov: The Elder Care Locator is a nationwide, directory assistance service designed to help older persons and caregivers locate local support resources for aging Americans. Toll free number (800) 677-1116.

www.eldersguild.org: The Elder's Guild is a CA-based non-profit dedicated to creating communities that re-image old age.

www.ioaging.org: The Institute on Aging is a CA-based non-profit dedicated to preserving the dignity, independence, and well-being of aging adults and people living with disabilities.

www.laughteryoga.com: Club founded by a doctor from India who was inspired by his research on the healing benefits of laughter.

www.lbda.org: The Lewy Body Dementia Association (LBDA) is a nonprofit organization dedicated to raising awareness of the Lewy body dementias (LBD), supporting people with LBD, their families and caregivers and promoting scientific advances

www.leadingage.org: Leading Age is a not-for-profit organization whose mission is to be the trusted voice for aging.

http://med.stanford.edu/letter: The letter project at Stanford was created to make end of life decisions an easier process for patients through a simple preformatted letter to your doctor.

www.pioneernetwork.net: The Pioneer Network is a not-for-profit organization dedicated to promoting culture change.

ABOUT THE AUTHOR

MARY ANN KONARZEWSKI, CMT, CMLDT, has worked with elders in long-term care for nearly two decades as an activity specialist, director, coordinator, consultant, and certified massage therapist. She is part of the wellness programs at Atria Valley View, Byron Park, and Moraga Post-Acute Care in the San Francisco Bay Area. She is the founder and principal of Heart Song, a private practice dedicated to enriching the lives of elders through creative expression, massage therapy, and other forms of engagement that facilitate more joyful, inspired, peaceful, and purposeful living. She works with individuals, families, elder care professionals, and long-term care communities, facilitating workshops for staff. She also conducts workshops for elders which include using acupressure for pain management, aromatherapy, celebrating individual lives, dreams, and artistic accomplishments, writing autobiography, and wisdom and gratitude circles. She is a published author and poet. For more information on her work, please see her websites at www.heartsongelders.com and www.heartsongmassage.abmp.com.

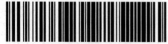

Made in the USA
San Bernardino, CA
10 November 2017